Eat Right for Life
with a Plant-Based Diet

The Secret to Permanent Weight Loss
and Optimal Health

Susan Allocco

Cover design by Michelle M. White
www.mmwgraphicdesign.com
Edited by Audra Gerber http://mycreativedetail.com

To contact the publisher, visit
www.createspace.com
To contact the author, visit
www.livingwellhealthcoach.com

ISBN: 978-1546645924
ISBN: 1546645926

Printed in the United States of America

CONTENTS

To my parents, who instilled in me at an early age the knowledge that there are only two things in life that are important: good health and happiness.

Introduction

I've enjoyed the benefits of a vegetarian diet for over 15 years, but it hasn't been without its challenges. I, like most people, made the assumption that a strict, plant-based diet ensures better health and weight loss. To be clear, it does, *but only when done correctly*.

When I initially transitioned, I jumped head-first into the diet. I immediately gave up all chicken, fish, and meat, and dined exclusively on processed vegetarian foods (frozen), mock meats, high-starch vegetables and grains, pasta, and other products made with wheat. I did not know about the danger of eating this way. As a result, I started to experience digestive problems and even put on weight. Through research and experimentation with my diet, I learned what went wrong and, more importantly, how to fix it.

I've written this book so that you do not make the same mistakes, and you can develop a plant-based diet that ensures optimal health and natural weight loss starting from day one of your transition. While the focus of this book is on a strict, plant-based diet, the information presented can help anyone, regardless of whether they're a flexitarian, vegan, or anything in between.

The diet encouraged in this book is not a fad diet. You'll learn how to eat right for the rest of your life. As you start to focus on the quality of the food that you eat, instead of the number of calories, the excess weight will fall off slowly, steadily, and permanently, and you'll feel great. I take a holistic approach, so you'll also learn about other lifestyle changes that can significantly impact your health and weight.

Think of this book as a road map to living well and being happy, because your diet and lifestyle have just as much of an impact on your emotional well-being as they have on your physical health.

Part 1

Why a Plant-Based Diet

"Nothing will benefit human health and increase the chances for survival of life on earth as much as the evolution to a vegetarian diet."

—Albert Einstein

Chapter 1

Plant-Based Defined

As you will soon learn, a plant-based diet is part of a healthy lifestyle. While my personal preference is vegetarian, a vegetarian or vegan diet may not work for you. If that turns out to be the case, included below are additional options that may be better.

Vegan

Vegan is the most restrictive and difficult to maintain. Vegans exclude meat, fish, poultry, and *all* animal-derived foods—including honey, eggs, and dairy—from their diet.

Vegetarian

Vegetarians don't eat meat, fish, or poultry but *will* consume animal-derived products. <u>The majority of studies in this book are based on a vegetarian diet.</u>

Pescatarian

This is a basic vegetarian diet with the addition of fish or a high-quality, fish oil supplement. I believe this may be a better option for children and older adults. Fish, or a fish oil supplement, provides fatty acids needed for proper brain development in children and numerous heart health benefits for older adults (see Chapters 2 and 9).

Flexitarian

The broadest category of plant-based diets is the flexitarian. Those on a flexitarian diet still eat meat, fish, and poultry, but only in *limited* amounts —i.e., no more than 20 to 25 percent animal protein. For this option to be a healthy one, it's important that you consume only free-range, organic poultry; grass-fed beef; and wild-caught fish with the least amount of mercury (see Chapter 2, "Fewer Toxins").

Regardless of which option you choose, if you commit to the dietary changes discussed in this book, you can expect to experience the following:

1) Natural weight loss without fad diets or calorie counting.
2) Support for a healthy immune system to protect you from illnesses and diseases.
3) More and longer-lasting energy.
4) A healthier outlook and renewed sense of well-being.

Chapter 2

The Undeniable Benefits

A Healthier You

There are loads of benefits for kicking the meat habit, especially when it comes to your health. When a vegetarian diet is compared with the standard American diet (SAD), those on the vegetarian diet develop fewer diseases, including heart disease, hypertension, obesity, type 2 diabetes, diet-related cancers, and diverticulitis.[1]

Less Heart Disease

A study of 27,529 Seventh-day Adventists (a vegetarian, Protestant sect) and meat eaters shows a definite link between meat consumption and heart disease.[2] The participants were tracked for 20 years, and the meat eaters had a 50 percent increase in the risk of coronary heart disease (CHD).

There were other studies with similar results. Five of these studies show that when compared to regular meat eaters, death from heart disease was lower on a plant-based diet as follows[3]:

> 34% lower in vegetarians
> 34% lower in pescatarians
> 26% lower in vegans
> 20% lower in flexitarians

As you can see, the vegetarians and pescatarians had the best results. I can't say for sure why the vegetarians did better than the vegans, but there is a scientific explanation why the pescatarians had such a low rate of CHD. The omega-3 DHA and EPA fatty acids, found in fish, are well known for their heart health benefits (see Chapter 9).

Lower Blood Pressure and Cholesterol

Transitioning to a vegetarian diet significantly lowers blood pressure. This was shown in several studies that included individuals with and without hypertension before they transitioned to the vegetarian diet.[4-8]

Other studies have proven that vegetarians have much lower cholesterol levels than meat eaters.[9-12]

Lower Risk of Cancer

We now know that diet is a stronger predictor of whether or not a person develops cancer than genetics.[13] Several studies show that cancer rates for vegetarians, in particular, are 25 to 50 percent lower than population averages.[14] One of the studies indicates that significant amounts of fruits and vegetables decrease cancers of the lung, breast, colon, bladder, stomach, mouth, larynx, esophagus, pancreas, and cervix.[15] What makes all these studies so relevant is that they controlled for smoking, body mass index, and socioeconomic status.

Fruits, vegetables, grains, legumes, and nuts, which are abundant in vegetarian and vegan diets, have high levels of phytochemicals. It's believed that phytochemicals protect us from both heart disease and cancer.[16] Plant-based diets are also the highest in fiber and beta-carotene, which also protect against cancer, especially colon cancer.[17]

But it's not just what you add to your diet that's important; it's also what you eliminate that plays a significant role in cancer prevention. In 2015, the World Health Organization (WHO) confirmed that consuming animal protein and dairy can increase your risk. They announced that processed meats, including bacon and sausages, cause cancer and that processed red meat probably does too. This conclusion came from a panel of 22 international experts who reviewed decades of research that included studies on human diet and health, and animal experiments.

For those concerned about breast or prostate cancer, the WHO also reported that dairy increases the production of the hormone insulin-like growth factor (IGF-1). Higher levels of IGF-1 cause higher levels of estrogen in women and higher levels of testosterone in men. Elevated levels of estrogen in women are responsible for breast cancer, and higher levels of testosterone in men can cause prostate cancer.[18]

Better Moods

Is it possible that vegetarians are happier than meat eaters? According to some studies, the answer is yes. In one study, researchers used three groups of individuals: 1) omnivores who ate meat, fish, and poultry daily; 2) a group who ate fish three to four times a week; and 3) a vegetarian group. The mood scores for the vegetarian group improved significantly after only two weeks.[19] For the omnivores and fish eaters, there was no change in their mood score.

The results of the study seem counterintuitive. Vegetarians get a significantly lower amount of omega-3 EPA (eicosapentaenoic acid) and DHA (docosahexaenoic acid) fatty acids from their diets. These fatty acids are essential for emotional health, but the only direct source is fish and fish oil (see Chapter 9). So, while the pescatarians in the study had a higher intake of EPA and DHA, the vegetarians still had better moods.

Sustainable Weight Loss

Most people assume that they'll lose weight by transitioning to a vegetarian diet, and studies seem to confirm it. In fact, several have shown that vegetarians in Western populations weigh less and have a lower body mass index (BMI) than meat eaters.[20, 21] (BMI is a measure of body fat based on height and weight.)

In one study that used a large group of vegetarians, the mean BMI was highest in meat eaters, lowest in vegans, and intermediate in vegetarians and fish eaters.[22] For the groups that did not eat meat, the mean BMI was the lowest for those individuals who stuck with the diet for five or more years.[23]

But the good news ends there. Contrary to these studies, adopting a strict, plant-based diet—vegetarian or vegan—does not guarantee weight loss. Many individuals give in to eating an unhealthy diet overloaded with grains, added sugar and processed foods (see Chapters 5 and 12 for more).

Fewer Toxins

Another health advantage of a strict, plant-based diet is the elimination of animal proteins that are high in antibiotics, hormones, and chemical toxins. Chemical toxins are a danger to your health and also interfere with weight loss by slowing down your metabolism.

Wild-caught fish contain dangerous mercury and PCBs (polychlorinated biphenyls). Unfortunately, farm-raised fish are not better, as they have a diet that consists of grains and legumes instead of their natural diet of 100 percent, omega-3 rich algae (see Chapter 9).

Most of the livestock and poultry consumed in the U.S. comes from factory farms. These animals are fed antibiotics to protect them from illnesses and diseases that would otherwise spread rapidly between animals because of the unsanitary, crowded living conditions. The problem with ingesting high levels of antibiotics is that the bacteria in your body become resistant to them, leaving you defenseless against the illnesses you may eventually need them for.

Pigs and poultry in factory farms are fed antimicrobials to control parasites and promote their growth. Some of the antimicrobials contain arsenic, a known human carcinogen.[24]

Cattle get injected with synthetic hormones to control their breeding and to make them gain weight. It's been suggested that these hormones are linked to the increased cancers in the U.S.

Less Inflammation and Oxidative Stress

Foods from animal sources contain advanced glycation end products (AGEs), especially when roasted, fried, or broiled.[25] AGEs promote oxidative stress that damages cells throughout the body. They also cause the inflammation linked to our diabetes and cardiovascular disease epidemics.[26]

The American Heart Association,[27] the American Institute for Cancer Research,[28] and the American Diabetes Association,[29] agree that you can significantly reduce AGEs by reducing solid fats (hydrogenated oil and animal fat), fatty meats, full-fat dairy products, and highly processed foods, and by increasing consumption of fish, legumes, vegetables, fruits, and whole grains.[30] These foods are low in AGEs even after you cook them.

Better Vision

A healthy plant-based diet is rich in fruits and vegetables, including those high in carotenoids. Carotenoids, especially lutein and zeaxanthin, are excellent for eyes. Spinach and collard greens are rich sources and are associated with a lower risk of age-related, ocular macular degeneration,[31] a common eye condition and a leading cause of vision loss for people who are 50 and older.

A Healthier Planet

The unsustainable demand for cheap animal protein has done and continues to do a tremendous amount of damage to our environment. Thankfully, the awareness of this problem has been growing, in large part, due to the public recognition by many environmental experts and organizations, including the World Health Organization (WHO) and the United Nations. It's this awareness that has created a growing number of vegetarians, vegans, flexitarians, and "meatless Monday" converts.

Keep in mind that the environmental effects detailed below do more than damage our planet; they're also a threat to your health, both directly and indirectly.

Water Pollution

Our rivers get contaminated from the runoff and sewage generated by factory farms where large numbers of livestock and poultry grow up in crowded, confined, and unsanitary facilities. The hormones and antibiotics that are given to livestock to keep them healthy, and to promote their growth, are excreted and end up in our water supply.[32]

Spills and leaks from waste-storage facilities and runoff from fields where excess amounts of animal waste are used as fertilizer contaminate both surface water and groundwater.[33]

How much waste is produced by factory-farmed animals? According to a report by the United States Senate Committee on Agriculture, Nutrition, and Forestry, they produce 130 times more waste than the entire human population—that's roughly five tons for every U.S. citizen. Some factory farms that have hundreds of thousands of animals produce as much waste as a town or a city.

Global Warming

Greenhouse gasses trap heat in the atmosphere and make the earth warmer. According to the U.S. Department of Agriculture, in 2012, the average American consumed 71.2 pounds of red meat and 54.1 pounds of poultry. The production needed to meet this demand created about 18 percent of worldwide greenhouse gasses. That's 5 percent more than the amount caused by transportation.[34]

Water Shortages

Raising all these animals, of course, requires a tremendous amount of water. One pound of processed beef, for example, requires 2,500 gallons of water. But just 250 gallons of water is used to grow one pound of soy.[35]

Dwindling Forests and Land Resources

Approximately 30 percent of the earth's entire land surface is now used to raise enough livestock to meet the demand for beef.[36] Forests continue to be cleared to create new pastures and to grow feed for livestock. The land erodes, and areas that were once fertile become deserts.

A World Health Forum report makes it clear that this will have a devastating impact on the not-too-distant future food supply.

"A rough calculation of current rates of soil degradation suggests we have about 60 years of topsoil left. Some 40% of soil used for agriculture around the world is classed as either degraded or seriously degraded – the latter means that 70% of the topsoil, the layer allowing plants to grow, is gone."—World Economic Forum

Part 2

Macronutrients: Protein, Fat, and Carbohydrates

"Macronutrients are nutrients that provide calories or energy and are required in large amounts to maintain body functions and carry out the activities of daily life."
—World Health Organization

Chapter 3

Protein:
Much Ado about Everything

When you transition to a strict, plant-based diet, it's important to focus on protein. Your body needs a nonstop supply of it to continuously build and repair cells,[1] break down food, and to grow and perform many other essential functions.[2]

Protein also plays a significant role in weight loss, metabolism, fat burning, muscle building, and stabilizing blood sugar. But not all proteins are the same. If you plan on starting a strict, plant-based diet, either vegetarian or vegan, you need to know what the differences are and how they can affect your body, mind, and moods.

All Proteins are NOT the Same

Each protein is made up of a group of amino acids connected in long chains; different proteins have various combinations of amino acids. A steak, for example, is made up of a different combination than a bean. Each amino acid plays a different role in your body. In other words, they have different benefits for your health.

Some are called nonessential amino acids, meaning your body can make them from other amino acids. The remainder are called essential amino acids, because you can only get them by eating certain foods.

Meat, poultry, fish, and eggs contain all of the essential and nonessential amino acids, so they're sometimes referred to as "complete" proteins. Most plant proteins are not considered complete, because they're missing one or more amino acids. This makes it important for vegetarians and vegans to get protein from a wide variety of plant sources throughout the day. By doing so, it will help ensure that you're getting all the essential amino acids (more on this later).

Protein's Role in Weight Loss and Maintenance

As mentioned earlier, protein plays a major role in weight loss. It reduces hunger, boosts your metabolism, optimizes HGH (human growth hormone) levels, and helps to burn fat and extra calories.

Reduces Hunger

Protein both satisfies[3] and reduces your hunger.[4] This is why it's important to have a quality protein with every meal.

Boosts Your Metabolism

Protein builds, repairs, and maintains muscles. And the more lean muscle you have, the higher your resting metabolism. Resting metabolism dictates how many calories your body burns while you're inactive (see Chapter 13).

Optimizes HGH for More Muscle and Less Body Fat

Several studies show that getting enough

protein in your diet optimizes HGH levels.[5] HGH is produced by the pituitary gland and is important to build and maintain muscle mass, burn fat, and increase resting metabolism. When we age, we naturally produce less HGH, which is why we get flabby and gain weight more easily.

Helps to Burn Fat Instead of Storing It

When the diet is high in carbohydrates, as is common in vegetarian and vegan diets, too much insulin, the fat-storage hormone, gets released (see Chapter 5). High-protein foods can help; they cause the hormone glucagon to be released, which stimulates fat burning instead of fat storage.[6]

Burns More Calories

The body needs to burn twice as many calories to digest protein than it does to digest carbohydrates or fats.[7] The fact is, more calories are burned to digest protein than any other food.

How Much Protein Is Enough?

Getting the right amount of protein is just as important as getting the right type. According to the USDA, you need the following amount each day[8]:

Adults and children over the age of four	50 g
Children under four	16 g
Lactating women	65 g

As you can see, the above recommendations do not take into consideration any other variables, like weight, calories consumed, or activity level. To account for these variables and get a more person-alized recommendation, you can use one of the following calculations:

Protein as a percentage of total calories and activity level.

The Institute of Medicine's recommendations are based on age, a percentage of total calories consumed, and activity level.

Age	Percentage of Calories Based on Activity Level
4–18 years of age	10–30%
19 years and older	10–35%

If you're over 19, you multiply the total amount of calories you consume in the average day by a number between 10 and 35 percent, which is dependent on your activity level. (Research confirms that protein requirements for athletes are higher than those for sedentary individuals.[9])

For example, if you consume around 2,000 calories a day and your activity level is average, the calculation is as follows:

2,000 calories X 0.15 = 300 calories of protein each day
Then convert calories to grams.
300 ÷ 4 = 75 grams of protein per day (one gram of protein equals four calories)

Protein as a percentage of weight and activity level.

For this method, the first step is to convert your weight from pounds to kilograms.

For example:

130 lbs. ÷ 2.2 = 59 kg
You then factor in your activity level.
59 kg X 0.8 * = 47 g of protein needed per day

* The average, nonathletic person needs approximately 8 percent of his body weight in protein. Depending on how athletic you are, you may need much more. If you're a vegetarian athlete, the American College of Sports Medicine (ACSM), the American Dietetic Association (ADA), and the Dietitians of Canada suggest that you consume 10 percent more protein.[10]

Best Protein Sources for a Plant-Based Diet

There are many plant proteins that make excellent replacements for animal protein. Some are comparable to animal proteins, as they provide all the essential and nonessential amino acids. The following are considered to be the best:

Legumes: Beans, Peas, and Lentils

Legumes, also known as "pulses," date back to 6000 BC. They're an essential part of a plant-based diet as well as diets in Mediterranean countries, India, Africa, Australia, the Middle East, and South America.

Legumes, which include beans, peas, and

lentils, do not have all the essential amino acids, but they have more protein than any other plant food. For example:

Legume	Protein per cup[11]
Lentils	17.86 g
Kidney beans	15.35 g
Black beans	15.24 g
Garbanzo beans	14.55 g
Pinto beans	15.41 g
Cannellini beans	16.06 g

Please note that the above is just a sampling. There are dozens of different types of legumes available, and each type has a unique nutritional value.

Legumes are high in fiber and essential nutrients, including folic acid, potassium, and B6. Legumes also contain potent antioxidants, flavonoids, and flavonols to protect against oxidative damage (free radicals that damage DNA, proteins, and membranes). It's no wonder they're heart healthy, lower cholesterol levels, and can even reduce the risk of many cancers.

Eggs

Eggs are considered a nearly perfect source of protein, as they're the most balanced and best source of all the essential amino acids.[12] There are 6.29 grams of protein per hard-boiled egg, and eggs are one of the few food sources of natural vitamin D.

If you're worried about cholesterol, don't be. It's no longer considered a concern as long you eat eggs in moderation. The Mayo Clinic now states that most healthy people can eat up to seven eggs a week with no increased risk of heart disease. The fact is, egg yolks do not raise cholesterol levels by more than 2 percent.[13] They contain choline, a vitamin-like nutrient that keeps the cholesterol moving through your bloodstream instead of accumulating on artery walls[14] (see Chapter 7). It's the high-sodium foods eaten along with the eggs—like bacon, sausages, and ham—that are now considered the real risk for heart disease.

Seeds

Seeds are an excellent part of any healthy diet and are particularly important for vegetarians and vegans. They contain healthy fats, nutrients, and protein. While there's a large variety to choose from, a strict, plant-based diet should include the three super seeds: chia, flax, and hemp.

Chia Seeds

Chia seeds are an energy powerhouse. They contain 4.4 grams of protein per ounce and have all the essential and nonessential amino acids.

It's not just their protein content that makes them an excellent addition to a plant-based diet; chia seeds are also high in antioxidants, calcium, magnesium, folate, fiber, and the essential fatty acid, omega-3 ALA (see Chapter 9).[15]

When placed in a liquid, chia seeds absorb it and expand. This creates a gelatin-like substance used as an egg replacement and thickener in vegan cooking.

Flaxseeds

With 5.1 grams of protein per ounce, flaxseeds are another great source of protein.

They're also a good source of manganese, folate, vitamin B6, magnesium, phosphorus, and copper, and are high in fiber.[16]

Like chia seeds, flaxseeds have lots of omega-3 ALA fatty acids, which, as you'll see in Chapter 9, are essential for good health. They have almost twice as much ALA as fish oil and have more lignans than any other plant food.[17] Lignans are phytochemicals that help lower LDL cholesterol (the bad one) and help provide protection against some cancers. A recent study showed <u>flaxseeds and its lignans were able to reduce the number and size of tumors and reduced metastasis by 45 percent.</u>[18]

Hemp Seeds

Hemp seeds may be the least known of the three super seeds, yet they've been used for thousands of years in traditional, oriental medicine.[19] As you can see from the chart below, hemp seeds have the most protein. Just one ounce has over 10 grams. That's more than ground meat has to offer, and it has all the essential and nonessential amino acids, making it a protein equal in quality to meat.

Hemp seeds are easy to digest and are an

exceptional source of nutrients, including manganese, phosphorus, vitamin B1 (thiamine), vitamin B3 (niacin), vitamin B5 (pantothenic acid), vitamin E, magnesium, and zinc. The oil from hemp seeds is the best plant source of omega-3 fatty acids (see Chapter 9).

Super Seed Protein Comparison[20]

	Per ounce	Per 100 g
Chia seeds	4.4 g	15.6 g
Flaxseeds	5.1 g	18.3 g
Hemp seeds (shelled)	10.3 g	36.7 g
Ground meat, 93% lean, broiled	7.43 g[21]	26.22 g[22]

Pseudograins

Pseudograins are frequently thought of as grains, but they're from a different family of plants. They include quinoa, amaranth, buckwheat, and wild rice. Quinoa, amaranth, and buckwheat contain all the essential amino acids, making them an excellent source of protein.

Pseudograins	Protein per cup (cooked)	Nutrients
Quinoa	8.1 g	Manganese, magnesium, iron, copper, zinc, and phosphorus.[23]
Amaranth	9 g	Magnesium, phosphorus, manganese and iron.[24] Also high in the amino acid lysine, [25] which is hard to find in plant foods.
Buckwheat	5.6 g	Manganese, magnesium, phosphorus, niacin, and zinc.[26]

Cheese

There's good news and bad news about cheese. First, the good news. Cheese is a complete protein, and there's lots of it (see below). It's also high in calcium, which is important to keep your bones strong.

Unfortunately, cheese and other dairy products contain an addictive protein called casein. It's similar to morphine and is right up there with sugar and wheat in terms of its ability to get you hooked.

If you go vegetarian or vegan, also consider that hard cheese is made with rennet, an enzyme from an animal's stomach. Some brands use vegetable rennet and will say so on the label.

	Protein per cup[27]
Cottage cheese (small curd)	25 g
Parmesan (grated)	28.42 g
Mozzarella (shredded)	24.83 g
Ricotta (whole milk)	27.70 g
Cheddar cheese (shredded)	25.84 g

Nuts

Nuts are rich in protein and are a staple in a healthy plant-based diet. The three nuts with the most protein are almonds (6.02 grams per ounce), dry-roasted pistachio nuts (5.94 grams per ounce), and walnuts (4.3 grams per ounce). Nuts are also heart healthy. They contain healthy, monounsaturated fats, packed with nutrition, including vitamin E, B6, folic acid, niacin, and minerals. And, contrary to what most people think, nuts have been proven to help with weight loss.[28]

Microalgae

Spirulina, a blue-green algae, and chlorella —a freshwater, green algae—are the richest plant sources of protein, provitamin A, and chlorophyll.[29] They have three times more protein than beef (just one teaspoon has the equivalent of one ounce of beef) and are much easier to digest.[30]

Additional health benefits include the following:

- Spirulina and chlorella are rich in chlorophyll, a green pigment that cleans and purifies the blood.

- Both help balance blood sugar (see Chapter 5).

- Chlorella is one of the most potent, natural detoxifiers. Its cell wall binds to heavy metals, environmental toxins, and PCBs, and then eliminates them from the body—necessary for better health and weight loss, as toxins can slow down your metabolism.

- Chlorella has a substance called Chlorella Growth Factor (CGF) that helps heal injuries and helps children grow.

- Spirulina is anti-inflammatory. It's one of the richest sources of gamma linoleic acid (GLA), an excellent anti-inflammatory (see Chapter 9).

- Both chlorella and spirulina contain nucleic acids needed for cell growth, repair, and renewal.

Protein Combinations

You don't need to eat plant proteins that contain all the essential and nonessential amino acids. If you combine certain incomplete plant proteins, you can get all the essential amino acids. For example, rice and beans are both incomplete proteins. Beans lack enough of the amino acid methionine, but grains have lots of it. Together they create a high-quality protein that's just as good as the protein in meat, eggs, and dairy.[31]

In addition to combining a whole grain with a legume, mixing nuts or seeds with legumes also gives you a complete, high-quality protein. You do not have to eat these protein combinations at the same meal, just sometime during the same day. That's one of the reasons why it's important for vegetarians and vegans to plan out their meals in advance.

> "You do not need to eat essential and nonessential amino acids at every meal, but getting a balance of them over the whole day is important."—University Maryland Medical Center

If you do wish to combine these proteins at the same meal, here are just a few ideas:

- Oatmeal topped with walnuts
- Hummus (garbanzo beans with sesame seed sauce)
- Lentils and almonds
- Pasta with peas
- Bean soup with blue corn chips
- Brown rice and beans
- Brown rice noodles with peanut sauce

The Best and Worst Meat Substitutes

Tempeh, fermented tofu, and seitan are meat replacements that can give you more variety and protein on a plant-based diet. Once you get the knack of cooking with these substitutes, you'll find it easy to swap out the meat in many recipes with one of them.

Seitan

Seitan is seasoned wheat gluten. It's a commonly used meat replacement in the Middle and the Far East, and has been around for hundreds of years. Seitan's texture is as close to meat as you can get with a plant protein. For this reason, it's called wheat meat and is popular in vegan and vegetarian restaurants. Seitan is versatile and also easy to use at home to replace beef, veal, or chicken in your recipes.

Just 3.5 ounces has around 16 grams of protein—almost two times the amount contained in tofu. It contains all the essential and nonessential amino acids but is low in the amino acid lysine. To create a better-balanced amino acid profile, seitan is usually seasoned with lysine-rich soy sauce when it's made.

Unfortunately, there are some issues with gluten and, therefore, seitan, so don't eat it frequently. It's hard to digest, can cause overeating, and may be addictive (see Chapter 5). Some individuals also have a sensitivity to gluten or, worse, have celiac disease, a severe genetic autoimmune disorder where the consumption of gluten causes damage to the small intestine. Whether you have a sensitivity to gluten or celiac disease, you should avoid seitan entirely.

That means you also need to be vigilant when dining out in vegetarian and vegan restaurants. As I mentioned, seitan is frequently used, but it usually does not say so on the menu. When you see "mock duck," for example, you can be relatively confident it's seitan. Be sure to ask.

Tempeh

Tempeh is an excellent meat substitute. It's made with soybeans that have been fermented with a mold, mixed with another whole grain—like brown rice, barley, or millet—and formed into a firm cake.

It's a nutritious, complete protein, comparable to meat, with all the essential and nonessential amino acids. There are 16 grams of protein in just three ounces.

The health benefits of tempeh include lower cholesterol and increased bone density. Studies show that the fermentation process increases the amount of riboflavin, vitamin B6, nicotinic acid (niacin), and pantothenic acid in tempeh. The process also eliminates all of the problems associated with unfermented soy products, which are discussed below.

Tofu

Tofu, which originated in China over a thousand years ago, is the most popular meat substitute in the West. You can find it in just about any conventional grocery store.

Also known as bean curd, tofu is made by curdling soy milk and pressing the curds into a cake. And, like other soy products, tofu is a complete protein. Three ounces of extra-firm tofu has 9 grams of protein.

For many years tofu has been touted as a health food because of the low cancer rate in Asia where soy is a staple food. But in Asia, unlike the

U.S., the soy products they consume are fermented, like tempeh, fermented tofu, miso, soy sauce, and nattō. It's the fermentation process that turns soy into a healthy food as the process eliminates most of its phytic acid. Phytic acid is a harmful substance that interferes with the absorption of key minerals, including calcium, zinc, magnesium, and iron.

The fermentation process also makes tofu easier to digest. Unfermented soy contains substances that block digestion. Fermentation neutralizes these substances[32] (see Chapter 8 for more). Unfortunately, fermented tofu is hard to find in the U.S.

There are other health issues associated with unfermented soy. Ninety percent of soy is genetically modified, and it contains high levels of aluminum, which is toxic to the immune system.[33] Eating too much of it may cause infertility, hypothyroidism, thyroid cancer, breast cancer, and kidney stones.[34]

There are 170 scientific studies that confirm the potential harm in consuming soy, but most Americans unknowingly eat it every day[35] as 60

percent of all processed and packaged foods contain soy by-products (see Chapter 12).

Chapter 4

Fat: Your Unexpected Ally

Fat has become the most misunderstood part of our diet. For years it's been demonized, particularly saturated fat, as the cause of heart disease and obesity. Yet the right dietary fat is key to good health and even weight loss. Healthy dietary fats

- Speed up your metabolism, reduce hunger, and stimulate fat burning[1];
- Help keep blood sugar stable (see Chapter 5), which reduces cravings and overeating;
- Are needed for cell membranes, the nervous system, and the immune system, and to make certain hormones[2];
- Keep skin and hair radiant, and help keep us "regular"[3];

- Provide twice as much energy as carbohydrates and burn slower for longer-lasting energy[4]; and
- Are needed to absorb the fat-soluble vitamins A, D, E, and K.

So, what about all the negative claims? It turns out that the real culprits are sugar and refined carbohydrates. They cause high cholesterol and triglycerides, and are responsible for our epidemic of obesity, type 2 diabetes, and heart disease.[5]

There are many different types of fat. While some are healthy, some will most definitely do damage.

Fats to Welcome into Your Diet

Medium-chain fats (MCFs) are some of the superstars of fats. MCFs have loads of benefits; they raise your metabolism, promote weight loss, and enhance fat burning and stamina.[6] These advantages are well known to many bodybuilders and athletes, and have been confirmed by studies.[7]

MCFs include butter and coconut oil, which is now considered a superfood. Dr. David Perlmutter, a brain-health expert, includes coconut oil as one of his recommendations to prevent Alzheimer's disease. It fuels the brain, fights inflammation, and fights off infections.

While both butter and coconut oil are saturated fats, current research has found that, in moderation, saturated fats are not harmful to heart health.[8,9] In fact, dietary saturated fat was a regular part of the standard American diet (SAD) before 1970, a time when obesity and type 2 diabetes were uncommon.[10] Keep in mind that most of the saturated fat in the SAD comes from animal protein, particularly red meats. By eliminating these proteins, it leaves room in your diet to add even more healthy fats.

Monounsaturated fats (MUFAs) are also healthy and should be a part of your diet. Contrary to popular belief, research has confirmed that eating more of these fats, along with a diet that minimizes sugar, actually promotes weight loss.

Monounsaturated fats include:

• Avocados

- Olives and olive oil
- Nuts and seeds, and their butters, like almond butter
- Walnut and macadamia oils
- Flaxseed and hemp seed oils
- Pumpkin seed oil

Cooking with Oils

The monounsaturated oils listed above have low burning, or smoke, points, so that at high temperatures, they get damaged molecularly and become hazardous to your health. Except for olive oil, use them in dips and salad dressings only.

If you cook with olive oil, which is popular in Mediterranean cooking, be sure to keep the temperature below the smoking point—low to medium-low temperatures on the stove.

Coconut oil, an MCF, has a high smoke point making it an excellent choice for high-heat cooking, like stir-fry recipes.

Fats to Kick to the Curb

Consuming any heated vegetable oil can

cause health issues, especially hydrogenated and refined oils. Problems include the build-up of toxins in the body and heart disease.

Vegetable oils and partially hydrogenated oils are found in abundance in processed foods. (For more good reasons to give them up, see Chapter 11.) The partially hydrogenated oils, also known as trans-fats, are used to extend the foods' shelf life. Fortunately, the Food and Drug Administration (FDA) has banned it, and food companies have three years from the time of this writing to eliminate it from all of their products.

Hydrogenated and refined vegetable oils include:

- Corn oil
- Safflower oil
- Canola oil
- Soybean oil
- Partially hydrogenated oils

How Much Fat Is Right for You

Getting the right fats into your diet is key to good health, but at what point does it become too much of a good thing? The answer is, it depends on how many carbohydrates you consume, your age, and how active you are.

In general, you can consume between 10 and 30 percent of your total calories in fat. The higher your consumption of carbohydrates (grains and sugars), the less fat you can eat, because when you consume both carbohydrates and fat together, your body will choose to burn the carbohydrates for energy and store the fat.[11]

Dr. Dean Ornish, who advocates a vegetarian diet to reverse heart disease, recommends you get 10 percent of your daily calories from fat, which is approximately 20 to 25 grams for the average person. Ten percent is low, but his diet is high in grains (carbs). On the other end of the spectrum is the Paleo Diet. Paleos can consume as much as 30 percent of their calories from fat (without gaining weight), because this diet excludes most carbohydrates—i.e., grains, legumes, and most sugars—and is based instead on exclusively eating wild game, fish, nuts, and seeds.

An individual on a healthy vegetarian diet can consume between 15 and 20 percent of calories in healthy fats, assuming the person is limiting their consumption of grains and sugars (see Chapter 5).

Chapter 5

Carbohydrates:
It's Complicated

"Today, approximately half of all calories consumed by most Americans come from carbohydrates."—Centers for Disease Control

Ah, carbohydrates. That's where a lot of vegetarians and vegans get it wrong. There are different types of carbohydrates. Some are healthy, while others can make you fat and sick. Unfortunately, most strict, plant-based diets are loaded with both. To develop a healthy diet, it's important to understand the different types of carbs and which ones you should avoid or minimize in your diet. Some may surprise you.

As you probably know, there are simple and complex carbohydrates. Simple carbohydrates are added sugars and naturally occurring sugars (the natural sugars found in food). Fruit and milk contain simple carbohydrates that are naturally occurring. Added sugars include table sugar (sucrose) and other types of sugars that are added to foods and beverages.

Starch is the natural sugar found in vegetables, grains, and legumes. These are referred to as complex carbohydrates. Complex carbs are considered healthy, because they contain nutrients and fiber. The fiber slows down digestion, so it prevents blood sugar spikes and keeps you feeling full longer. But some complex carbs are what I call low-quality complex carbs. Whole wheat and most potatoes, for example, will spike your blood sugar as fast as table sugar (more on these low-quality complex carbs later).

In one respect, carbohydrates are all the same. When you eat any carbohydrate, your body converts it to glucose (sugar) and releases it into the bloodstream, which is why it's referred to as blood sugar. The body responds to blood sugar increases by producing the hormone insulin to move the sugar out of the blood and into your cells, where it can be used for energy or stored as fat to be used at another time for energy.

But different types of carbs affect blood sugar differently. Low-quality complex carbs and added sugars cause a quick spike in blood sugar and a rapid boost of energy. This is followed by a rush of insulin to get all of that sugar out of your bloodstream. Blood sugar levels crash and leave you foggy headed, tired and irritable. Naturally, you then crave more of these carbs to pick you back up again both physically and emotionally. This ongoing, vicious cycle eventually causes health issues, weight gain, and excess fat. Where that fat gets stored depends on the type of carb that you eat.

When you eat high-quality carbs, your blood sugar stays stable, or balanced, and amazing things happen as your body can start to burn fat instead of sugar for energy.[1] Fat gives you twice as much energy as carbohydrates, and it's a long-lasting, stable energy.[2] You also stop craving sweets and low-quality complex carbs, because you no longer need a carb "fix"; your memory and moods improve[3]; and you may even look younger.[4] Imagine, all of that in addition to losing weight and excess fat!

Now that you have an overview of the different carbohydrates, it's time to get down to the specifics.

STARCH: A Sticky Situation

As I stated earlier, starch is the natural sugar found in grains, legumes, and vegetables. Like all carbohydrates, it gets converted to blood sugar when you eat it. While foods with starch also contain vital nutrients and fiber, some are high in starch and should be eaten only in moderation. Potatoes and rice, for example, can spike your blood sugar "faster and higher than table sugar or candy.[5]" Sweet corn is no better; it has so much starch (40 percent) that eating it is like eating a doughnut.[6]

High-starch foods that should be eaten in moderation are the following:

Rice
Potatoes
Corn (Blue corn is better if you can find it.)
Beans
Peas
Wheat

Spelt

Amaranth

Note: Beans are an important staple in a vegetarian and vegan diet, because they're one of the best sources of protein (see Chapter 3). But their high starch content is one of the reasons you need to manage your carbohydrate consumption carefully (more on this later).

There are some things you can do to reduce the blood sugar spike you get from some popular, high-starch foods, specifically rice, potatoes, and pasta.

Rice: Starch is what makes rice (and other starchy foods) stick, so the stickier the rice, the more starch the rice contains. Choose non-sticky rice, like basmati, jasmine, and long-grain rice. Long-grain brown rice is a great choice; not only is it lower in starch, but it's also an excellent source of manganese, selenium, phosphorus, copper, magnesium, and niacin (vitamin B3).[7]

Potatoes: When it comes to starch, not all potatoes are created equal. It's best to choose new potatoes or waxy potatoes. They have a lower starch content and will not affect blood sugar as much as old potatoes (baking potatoes). Depending on the type of potato, a new potato can have up to one-half the amount of starch.

How you prepare potatoes can also lower its impact on your blood sugar. If you cook potatoes, refrigerate them for 24 hours, and then consume them (either cold or reheated), it reduces the blood sugar increase by 25 percent.[8]

Pasta: According to Dr. Denise Robertson, a senior nutrition scientist at the University of Surrey, the same blood-sugar-reducing technique also works for pasta. In a small study, researchers found that eating pasta that was chilled overnight led to a lower spike in blood sugar, but by cooking, cooling, and then reheating the pasta, it reduced blood sugar levels by 50 percent.[9]

The reduction in glucose is due to what's called "resistant starch." Resistant starch is increased by the process of heating, cooling, and reheating and is broken down by the body differently than starch. The body treats it more like fiber so that there's less glucose, insulin, and hunger, and ultimately, less fat storage. That does not mean you can eat all the potatoes and pasta that you want. You still have to carefully manage your carbohydrate consumption on a strict, plant-based diet. But, on those rare occasions when you do indulge, the resistant starch will at least provide you with more fiber and a somewhat healthier food.

Grains: Friend or Foe

Unlike whole grains, refined grains and their flours are made by a process that removes their nutrients and fiber. While some nutrients are added back in, the fiber is not, so they're digested quickly, cause blood sugar spikes, and should be avoided.

Whole grains, on the other hand, are highly valued in vegetarian and vegan diets. They contain all their natural nutrients and fiber, bulk up a meal, and add variety and protein (see Chapter 3, "Protein Combinations" for more). Unfortunately, eating excessive amounts of grains, a common mistake made by many vegetarians and vegans, can cause several problems, including mineral deficiencies, hormone imbalances, digestive problems, and fat accumulation in the most dangerous places.

Vegetarian and vegan diets can easily become overloaded with simple carbs and low-quality complex carbs from frequently eating sweets, pizza, pasta, and bread, and relying on recipes that use wheat and refined grains as the main component of the dish.

Mineral Deficiencies

A strict, plant-based diet contains many foods, including grains, which are high in phytic acid. Phytic acid is a substance that blocks the body's ability to absorb essential minerals, including zinc, calcium, and magnesium. It puts vegans and vegetarians, in particular, at risk for mineral deficiencies.[10] The phytic acid in just one bagel or sandwich, for example, reduces your body's ability to absorb magnesium by 60 percent.[11,12] Because of their phytic acid content, grains are the second-most common cause of iron-deficiency anemia after blood loss.[13]

Poor Digestion

In addition to creating mineral deficiencies, phytic acid also inhibits essential enzymes that are needed to digest food properly. These enzymes include pepsin[14] and trypsin,[15] which are necessary to break down proteins, and amylase[16] that's required to break down starch.

One way to tackle the phytic acid problem is to maintain a sufficient amount of healthy gut bacteria (see Chapter 8 for more).

Overeating

Lectin, a protein in wheat and other grains, including rye, barley, and rice, blocks the hormone leptin.[17] Leptin signals the brain that you're satisfied, so when leptin is blocked, you overeat.

Addiction

Gluten is a protein in many grains. It's what gives the dough its elastic texture. It's also what makes us happy—and addicted. Gluten triggers the release of exorphins that are similar to the feel-good endorphins that you get from exercise, especially running. Exorphins bind to the same brain receptors as opiate drugs[18] and create feelings of comfort and pleasure.[19,20] It's believed that it's the addictive nature of grains that has made them into the primary food source that they are today.[21]

Many people also find gluten hard to digest or have a sensitivity to it. If you're one of them, you may feel tired and agitated, and experience bloating, gas, and bowel trouble.[22] In either case, it's best to remove all of it from your diet.

Grains that contain gluten include the following: *

Barley
Bulgur
Couscous
Dinkel (wheat, spelt)
Durum (type of wheat used mainly for pasta)
Einkorn (primitive, small-grained wheat of Europe and Asia)
Farina (a hot wheat cereal)
Farro (another name for wheat)
Fu (dried gluten used in Japanese cooking)
Freekeh (Middle Eastern wheat cereal)
Graham flour (can be made from wheat or chickpeas)
Kamut (type of wheat)
Khorasan (ancient variety of wheat)
Matzo, matzah (traditional Jewish, unleavened wheat bread)
Mir (a cross between wheat and rye)
Rye (a type of wheat) **

Seitan (pure wheat gluten used in vegetarian, vegan, and Indonesian dishes)
Semolina (type of wheat used mainly for pasta)
Spelt (ancient wheat, includes dinkel and farro) **
Triticale (hybrid cross of wheat and rye)
Wheat

* From the Celiac Support Association®

** Rye and spelt are mainly used for baking and are low in gluten.

Gluten-free grains include oats, teff, (a mineral-rich grain), millet (high in B vitamins, magnesium, and tryptophan), and rice.

The Case Against Wheat

Of all the grains, wheat is the worst, and not just refined wheat. Whole wheat is one of the low-quality complex carbs I mentioned earlier. The complex carbohydrate in whole wheat has a unique structure called amylopectin A. This structure makes whole wheat quick and easy to digest,[23] which is why it increases blood sugar higher than almost any other type of simple or complex carbohydrate.[24,25]

> Eating just two slices of whole wheat bread is the equivalent of eating two tablespoons of table sugar.

A Top Addictive Food

Wheat is one of the top three addictive foods (the other two are sugar and cheese). How do you know that you're hooked?

Products made from wheat affect you in many of the same ways that a drug affects an addict. For example:

- The idea of giving it up makes you upset.[26]
- You frequently have intense cravings for foods made with it.
- When you try to give it up, you have withdrawal symptoms (see Chapter 6).[27]

Other clues that you're addicted are the following:

- Although you're no longer hungry, you keep eating it.[28]

- You have one or more of the allergy symptoms listed below,[29] which clear up when
you totally eliminate wheat from your diet.[30]

> Heartburn
> Headache
> Irritability or nervousness
> Joint pain
> Unexplained weight gain

Visceral Fat

Some vegetarians are thin but carry around
what Dr. William Davis has coined a "wheat belly."
When you eat a lot of wheat, common with vegans
and vegetarians, it causes fat, known as visceral fat,
to accumulate around the abdomen and internal
organs. There are many health issues associated
with visceral fat, including inflammation, cancer,
autoimmune disorders, and brain disease.[31] It can
also slow down your metabolism and cause you to
gain even more weight.[32]

Hormone Imbalances

Visceral fat affects the hormones estrogen,
testosterone, and prolactin. In men, visceral fat
converts testosterone to estrogen, resulting in too

much estrogen and too little testosterone.[33] That can cause infertility, weight gain, a loss of muscle mass, and overly sensitive men. Prolactin, a hormone responsible for breast growth, also increases. [34,35] It's the high prolactin combined with the high estrogen that causes men to grow large breasts.[36]

In women, visceral fat increases testosterone, estrogen, and prolactin. More estrogen and prolactin cause larger breasts and also increase the risk of breast and endometrial cancer.[37,38] Too much testosterone in women is responsible for unwanted facial hair, thicker mustaches, male pattern baldness, and possibly polycystic ovary syndrome (PCOS) that can cause infertility.[39]

A Healthier Alternative: Pseudograins

Pseudograins are a great alternative to grains. While they may look like grains, they're biologically different. Pseudograins are gluten-free, nutritious, and high in protein and fiber, and are a good addition to a strict, plant-based diet (see Chapter 3). They include:

Quinoa
Amaranth
Buckwheat

Wild rice

Surprisingly, wild rice is not a "rice"; it's an aquatic *grass*. It's rich in minerals, B vitamins, and the amino acid lysine. In addition to being more nutritious than traditional grains, wild rice is a hardy plant, so they rarely treat it with pesticides.[40]

Please note that while these pseudograins are gluten-free, they still contain phytic acid, which interferes with the absorption of essential minerals.

The Sour Truth about Sugar

Sugar is a simple carbohydrate and includes both added sugars and the naturally occurring sugars found in fruit and dairy.

Added Sugar: Your #1 Enemy

Added sugar is finally getting credit for the damage that it does to our health: It causes excess fat, weight gain, and—according to numerous studies—serious health issues, including cancer.

The American Heart Association recommends that women consume no more than six teaspoons (24 grams) of added sugar per day and that men consume no more than nine teaspoons (36 grams).[41] Six and nine teaspoons, respectively, is still too much, yet we consume a lot more than that.

In fact, the average American eats or drinks the equivalent of 22 teaspoons of sugar a day, and children aged 14 to 18 consume a whopping 34 teaspoons.[42] Vegetarians, vegans, and flexitarians are no exception; they eat just as much sugar as the average omnivore.[43]

If you consume a lot of added sugars and have tried to stop, you already know how difficult it is. We now know why. Studies show that sugar is four times more addictive than cocaine[44] and is just as addictive as heroin.[45] When you eat sugar your brain releases endorphins that reduce anxiety, give you a sense of well-being, and temporarily boost your self-esteem. Sugar also triggers the brain to release serotonin that acts as an antidepressant.[46] It's easy to understand why we reach for sweets when we're stressed out or unhappy.

> *"Our findings clearly demonstrate that intense sweetness can surpass cocaine reward, even in drug-sensitized and addicted individuals."*[47]

Most people don't realize just how much sugar gets added to their diets via the consumption of processed foods and beverages. Of the 600,000 food items in America, it's estimated that a whopping 80 percent contain added sugar. Even the most unlikely products have it, like ketchup, yogurt, and tomato sauce.

If you read product labels, it's still hard to know how much sugar has been added, due to a technique used by food companies called "ingredient splitting." They display the ingredients in descending order, from ingredients with the most weight on top to those with the least weight on the bottom. So, instead of using one type of added sugar, which would cause it to appear on top, they use several different kinds (or names) so that these sugars are lower down on the list. Not only does it make the product appear to have much less sugar than it has, but it elevates the healthier ingredients to the top, making the food appear much healthier than it is.[48]

When reading food labels, remember that every 4 grams of sugar = 1 teaspoon of table sugar.

Different names and types of sugars that you'll see on food labels include:

Agave nectar

Anhydrous dextrose (powdered dextrose)

Beet sugar

Brown sugar

Cane crystals

Cane juice

Cane sugar

Corn sweetener

Corn syrup (High-fructose corn syrup)

Coconut palm sugar

Confectioner's powdered sugar

Crystal dextrose

Crystalline fructose

Dextrose

Evaporated cane juice

Evaporated corn sweetener

Fructose

Fruit juice concentrates

High-fructose corn syrup (HFCS)

Honey

Lactose

Liquid fructose

Invert sugar

Maltose

Malt syrup

Maple syrup

Molasses

Nectars (e.g., peach or pear)

Raw sugar

Rice syrup or brown rice syrup

Sorghum

Sucrose

Syrup

Turbinado

White granulated sugar

Food labeling laws complicate the issue even more, because they do not require companies to differentiate between the added sugars and naturally occurring sugars. Therefore, the total carbohydrates shown on the label includes all added sugars plus the fructose or lactose found naturally in fruits and milk.

> On the product label, Total Carbohydrates - Fiber = Net Carbohydrates (all added sugars + naturally occurring sugars)

The only way to eliminate these sugars from your diet is to give up processed foods, soft drinks, and fruit juices, including the "all natural" ones (see Chapter 12).

A Healthier Way to Add Sweetness

There are some natural alternatives to table sugar. Some are safe, even for those with type 2 diabetes, but others spike blood sugar levels just like table sugar.

Raw honey, coconut sugar, maple syrup, and date sugar are popular. These natural sweeteners have some nutritional value and add a great taste. But they can still spike your blood sugar, so it's best to use these sweeteners infrequently and in small amounts.

A better choice is a sugar alcohol (a hybrid of sugar and alcohol), preferably xylitol*. Made from birch bark, xylitol won't spike your blood sugar.

And it has a unique benefit: It's been proven to stop the formation of cavities.[49]

Another good option is stevia, which they make from a natural herb that grows in South America. Like xylitol, it works well in beverages and recipes, and will not impact blood sugar. Look for a USDA organic brand to ensure that it's pure. Keep in mind that regardless of what type of sweetener you choose, if you use it frequently, it trains your taste buds to prefer sweeter foods.[50]

When it comes to artificial sweeteners, your best bet is to avoid them. Artificial sweeteners give us the sweet taste that we like, without the spike in blood sugar and calories. But there's a big down-side: Research shows that artificial sweeteners stimulate the appetite, promote fat storage, cause weight gain, and increase cravings for carbs. In one study using rats, those fed artificial sweeteners consumed more calories and gained more weight than rats fed foods sweetened with sugar.[51] Artificial sweeteners have also been linked to several health concerns.

* Please note that xylitol, and any products made with it, is toxic to dogs.

The Dark Side of Naturally Occurring, Simple Sugars

The naturally occurring, simple sugars found in foods are fructose and lactose. Lactose is the sugar found in dairy products. Many people have a difficult time digesting lactose and have to eliminate it from their diets.

Fructose is the natural sugar in fruit, dried fruit, honey, and maple syrup. It's also in high-fructose corn syrup (HFCS); agave, a natural sweetener; and refined, added sugars (also known as sucrose and table sugar).

Refined, added sugars	50% fructose
High-fructose corn syrup	55% fructose
Agave	70 to 90% fructose depending on brand

According to the Third National Health and Nutrition Examination Survey, fructose consumption in the U.S. has more than doubled in the last 30 years and is five times higher than it was 100 years ago.[52] This overconsumption comes from eating refined, added sugars and high-fructose corn syrup,[53] both of which are in many processed foods and beverages (see Chapter 12).

Too much fructose in the diet creates several issues; it turns to fat rapidly, makes you overeat, creates visceral fat, and ages you faster.

Turns to Fat Quickly

The body metabolizes fructose differently than other sugars. Just about every cell in the body can break down glucose for energy. Fructose, on the other hand, goes right to the liver, where it gets converted to fat quickly.

When there's too much fructose in the diet, fat accumulates in the liver cells, a condition called nonalcoholic fatty liver disease. If it's not reversed early on, it can lead to scar tissue and eventually a liver that no longer functions properly.[54]

Makes You Overeat

If your diet is consistently high in fructose, it can cause leptin resistance.[55] Leptin is the hormone that sends a signal to the brain that you're full. When your system is frequently bombarded with leptin, you develop a resistance to it. That means that while your body is producing enough, your brain no longer receives the message to stop eating.

Causes Visceral Fat

Just like wheat, fructose produces visceral fat. And, as you know by now, visceral fat is the dangerous fat that accumulates around your abdomen and internal organs, including your liver and heart. Fructose is worse than wheat. Studies now suggest that when you eat fructose along with a fat, or before a fat, that fat's more likely to be stored instead of burned for energy.[56]

Accelerates Aging

Fructose drives what's called the Maillard reaction seven times faster than glucose.[57] The Maillard reaction is a chemical reaction between an amino acid and sugar that produces advanced glycation end products (AGEs).

AGEs cause body cells to age faster and speed up degenerative processes like cancer.[58] They make skin more prone to sun damage, cause wrinkles by damaging the skin's elastin and collagen, and cause tissue decay,[59] stiff arteries, cataracts, cognitive decline, and dementia.[60]

May Affect Cardiovascular Health

While there is no definitive proof that too much fructose is bad for cardiovascular health, there seems to be some evidence of the following health issues[61]:

- Elevated triglycerides
- Increased LDL cholesterol (the bad one)
- Increased blood pressure
- Insulin resistance
- Production of more free radicals that damage DNA and cells

Fructose and Sucrose and Glucose, oh my!

Eliminating added sugars and managing grains to control your blood sugar is bar none the best way to protect your health.

Can Help Prevent Cancer

Conclusive evidence from many studies has proven that sugar is what feeds cancer cells. Below are just a few findings from various studies:

- Fructose causes pancreatic cancer tumors to grow more quickly. Anyone who wants to cut their risk of cancer should reduce the amount of sugar they eat.[62]

- Depriving cancer cells of glucose leads to cancer cell death.[63]

- Tumor cells use a lot more glucose than healthy cells. Research has demonstrated how this process takes place and how to stop it from controlling a tumor's growth.[64]

- There's a "straightforward and clear association between high-glycemic foods and the risk of colorectal cancers"—Simin Liu, MD, ScD, Brown University

- Cancers are so sensitive to the sugar supply that cutting that supply will suppress cancer.[65]

Optimizes Your Brain and Emotional Health

Consistently high levels of glucose and insulin every day can cause a decline in your memory and your ability to learn.[66] And, if you're susceptible to depression, grains can trigger it or make it worse.[67] Wheat and corn have been shown to reduce brain serotonin,[68] a natural mood regulator and antidepressant.

A Guideline to Managing Your Carb Load and Blood Sugar

Managing your carbohydrate consumption doesn't have to be complex. Below you'll find a clear guideline. If you stick with it, you'll eliminate blood sugar spikes and crashes, and experience more sustainable energy, weight loss, and overall good health.

Eliminate:

- Added sugars (particularly refined, added sugars, HFCS, and agave)
- Refined grains (products made with white rice and flour, including pasta and bread)
- Fruit juices *
- Processed foods (see Chapter 12)

Eat Sparingly:

- Dried fruit (All are high in fructose.)
- Whole wheat
- Honey (41% fructose) and maple syrup

Eat in Moderation:

- Whole grains (particularly those with gluten)
- Pseudograins
- High-starch vegetables (potatoes, yellow corn, beans, and peas)
- Fruits high in sugar (e.g., bananas, pineapples, mangoes, grapes, watermelon, dates, cherries, and apples)

Enjoy Lots Of:

- Leafy green vegetables (e.g., kale, spinach, arugula, Swiss chard, collard greens, romaine lettuce, and mustard greens)
- Cruciferous vegetables (e.g., broccoli, cabbage, and cauliflower)
- Low-starch vegetables (e.g., artichokes, asparagus, baby corn, peppers, mushrooms, and green, wax and Italian beans)
- Fruit low in sugar (Berries have the least amount of sugar.)

* Fruit juice is high in fructose. For example, 100 percent orange juice has 1.8 grams of fructose per ounce, while soda contains 1.7 grams per ounce.[69] What's more, there's no fiber to slow down its digestion.

You may find that initially counting carbs is helpful. If so, use the guideline below. But, keep in mind that everyone is different—e.g., different activity levels, age, weight, metabolism, and health issues, if any—so use it as a general guide only.

Over 150 grams of carbohydrates per day. This will cause most people to gain weight unless they're exceptionally active or an athlete.

100 to 150 grams per day. A healthy vegan or vegetarian diet will naturally fall within this range. If you are slim and active, it will allow you to maintain your current weight. If you're heavy and have no health issues, you should lose any excess weight.

50 to 100 grams per day. For the majority of vegans and vegetarians, this is too restrictive but doable and sustainable if you opt for a flexitarian diet. It's a good option for those individuals who are obese or have prediabetes or type 2 diabetes. In fact, The American Diabetes Association recommends approximately 55 to 60 grams of carbohydrates per day or around 15 grams per meal.

Additional Support to Help Balance Blood Sugar

Acidic foods, healthy fats, and certain minerals can help you keep your blood sugar balanced. Keep in mind, though, that these additions may only make a small difference and cannot replace the impact you'll have if you eliminate added sugars and manage your carbohydrate consumption.

Acidic Foods. Add vinegar (including apple cider vinegar) or lemon juice to foods and dressings.[70] An Italian study found that if a meal includes a dressing made with four teaspoons of vinegar and two teaspoons of oil, your blood sugar will be as much as 30 percent lower.[71]

That works great with high-starch foods, like potatoes. For example, if you make potato salad with vinegar and olive oil, the addition of the vinegar reduces the glycemic index (GI) of the potatoes by 25 percent.[72] The glycemic index (GI) ranks how quickly and high a particular food boosts sugar and insulin levels.

Healthy Fats. Cooking with a healthy fat, or adding it to food, will lower the food's GI[73,74] as the fat slows down the digestive process—i.e., the absorption of sugar into the bloodstream. Coconut oil is an excellent choice and is considered the best food for keeping blood sugar stable.

Chlorella. Chlorella is a freshwater, green algae that comes in tablet or powder form. Studies have found that chlorella reduces body fat, total serum cholesterol, and fasting blood glucose levels.[75] (This is your blood sugar level when you wake up, before you have anything to eat.)

Magnesium and Chromium. The minerals magnesium and chromium play a role in normalizing blood sugar levels.[76,77,78] Normalizing means they will raise or lower blood sugar depending on what your body needs at the time.

Foods high in chromium include broccoli (an excellent source), garlic, basil, apples, potatoes, green beans, and bananas.[79] Getting enough magnesium from food is much more challenging, especially for those on a plant-based diet that's high in grains. As I mentioned earlier, grains and legumes are high in phytic acid, a substance that interferes with the absorption of vital minerals, including magnesium (see Chapter 8 for help).

Chamomile Tea. Chamomile is a traditional herb that's been used for centuries. It's most commonly known as a sleep aid and for relieving upset stomachs. We now know that it also lowers blood sugar and blood pressure,[80] and helps thin the blood,[81] all of which could help decrease the risk of heart attacks and strokes.

Chapter 6

Withdrawal:
The Biggest Hurdle

Sugar and wheat are highly addictive, so when you stop eating them, your body reacts just as it would if you were withdrawing from an addictive drug.[1] The most common symptoms include headaches, jitteriness, fatigue, nausea, and depression.

The good news is, not everyone experiences withdrawal symptoms, and, if you do, they're short-lived. For most people, symptoms last only a couple of days. Once you get over this hurdle, you'll feel better than you have in quite some time. And you'll feel encouraged to make more healthy diet and lifestyle changes.

Of course, you have the option of eliminating them slowly. But this just extends the suffering; you'll be struggling with powerful cravings for a longer period and, as a result, will be more inclined to give up trying.

Below are some things you can do that may help with cravings and other withdrawal symptoms:

Increase serotonin, the feel-good neurotransmitter. Higher levels of serotonin help you sleep better, boost your mood,[2] and help with cravings.[3] Here are some simple ways to increase it:

- Get plenty of sun. Research shows that exposure to bright light increases serotonin levels.
- Supplement with Rhodiola and 5-HTP. Rhodiola is an adaptogenic herb that raises both serotonin levels and feel-good opioids, like beta-endorphins.[4,5]
- 5-Hydroxytryptophan (5-HTP) also increases the production of serotonin.[6]

Note: As you lose weight, serotonin levels drop and cause food cravings and low moods.[7]

Take magnesium and vitamin C. Magnesium deficiency is common and can increase some of the symptoms of wheat withdrawal.

Vitamin C supplementation also helps. Dr. Mark Hyman recommends 2,000 milligrams of buffered vitamin C once or twice a day to help relieve withdrawal symptoms.[8] That's high, so take this amount only during withdrawal and with the guidance of a holistic health practitioner or your physician.

Drink water. Get at least eight cups a day.

Use downtime to withdraw. Start the elimination on a quiet, long weekend when you have no commitments. Then relax doing something you enjoy—e.g., download some movies or read a good book.

Don't overexert yourself. Instead of a strenuous exercise routine (if that's what you normally do), take long, relaxing walks instead.

Sleep. Get at least eight hours of sleep, take naps if needed, and rest both physically and emotionally (see Chapter 10).

Part 3

Micronutrients: Vitamins, Minerals, and Fatty Acids

"Called micronutrients because they are needed only in minuscule amounts, these substances are the 'magic wands' that enable the body to produce enzymes, hormones and other substances essential for proper growth and development."

—World Health Organization

Chapter 7

Supplements: The Nonnegotiables

Taking the necessary dietary supplements is an essential step in transitioning to a strict, plant-based diet. It can make the difference between thriving physically and emotionally or feeling run down and unable to think clearly. When you give up meat, fish, and poultry, you're also losing the best, and sometimes the only, sources of vitamin B12, zinc, and iron. As you probably know by now, mineral deficiencies can also develop due to the high amount of phytic acid in grains and legumes.

To protect your good health and avoid nutrient deficiencies, the following supplements should be taken by vegetarians and vegans:

Supplement	Best Sources	Function
Vitamin B12	Meat and fish	Helps keep nerves and blood cells healthy. Helps make DNA, the genetic material in all cells. Prevents a type of anemia that makes people tired and weak.
Zinc	Red meat and shellfish	To grow, develop, and heal wounds. Needed by the immune system and for neurological function, taste, and reproduction.
Iron*	Beef, chicken, liver, clams, mussels, and oysters	Moves oxygen throughout the body. Needed to make red blood cells. Deficiency causes fatigue and effects brain function and immune system.

Magnesium	Pumpkin seeds, spinach, Swiss chard, soybeans, sesame seeds, quinoa, black beans, and cashew nuts	Needed by every organ in the body, especially the heart, muscles, and kidneys. Also needed for teeth, bones, energy production, heart health, and relaxation.
Probiotic	Fermented foods	Increases and maintains healthy intestinal flora, which neutralizes phytic acid for better absorption of essential minerals.[1] Creates B vitamins (see Chapter 8).
Multivitamin		To help combat potential mineral deficiencies due to the phytic acid in grains, legumes, nuts, and seeds.

| Choline | Meat, fish, chicken, wheat germ, eggs | A vitamin-like essential nutrient that regulates the homocysteine concentration in blood. Deficiency can cause nonalcoholic fatty liver disease and muscle damage. High levels can cause heart attacks and strokes.[2] **Only vegans** are at risk for a deficiency[3] and should be monitored periodically for a possible need to supplement. |

* Vegetarians and vegans need 1.8 percent more iron than carnivores, because the iron from plant sources is difficult to absorb.

Chapter 8

Microflora:
The Anti Antinutrient

As mentioned before, one of the biggest problems with vegetarian and vegan diets is the significant amount of phytic acid in the foods that are the mainstay of these diets.

Phytic acid is commonly referred to as an antinutrient, as it blocks the absorption of essential minerals, including zinc, calcium, magnesium, iron, and copper. To combat this issue, eat fermented foods and take a probiotic supplement.

There are two ways that fermented foods help. First, when food is fermented, the fermentation process significantly reduces the amount of phytic acid. Second, fermented foods are rich in good bacteria (also known as intestinal flora or gut microflora) that reside in the intestinal tract. Individuals with a healthy supply of good bacteria are not as affected by phytic acid, because the good bacteria produce phytase, an enzyme that neutralizes the phytic acid.[1]

Maintaining a healthy supply of gut flora also provides other important health benefits: It balances out bad bacteria to prevent diarrhea and infections, strengthens the immune system, and helps prevent food allergies and cancer.[2] In one study done by UCLA, the researchers found that probiotics also alter brain functions, supporting the belief that the "gut-brain connection is a two-way street.[3]"

"The regular intake of probiotic preparation may represent a cheap and safe tool in order to convert a diet with a low potential for bioavailability of trace minerals and proteins, such as the vegetarian diet, into a diet with a high bioavailability potential. The benefit of such an approach would not be restricted to vegetarians.[4]"

In addition to minimizing phytic acid and increasing good bacteria, there are other health benefits that come from fermentation:

- Makes food easier to digest as the protein gets predigested.
- Increases the food's nutritional value. Fermentation creates B vitamins (including folic acid, riboflavin, niacin, thiamin, and biotin).
- Helps rid the body of toxins, including heavy metals.
- Promotes a healthy digestive tract and immune system.

Some of the more well-known fermented foods include:

- Tempeh: fermented soy—an excellent source of protein
- Kefir: fermented milk
- Yogurt
- Sauerkraut *
- Kimchi: fermented cabbage or other vegetables and spices
- Soy sauce
- Pickled vegetables
- Vinegar
- Miso: fermented soy

- Some cheeses (Look for organic cheeses made from raw milk.)

  * Sauerkraut must be unpasteurized or the heat will kill the good, as well as the bad, bacteria.

  If you plan on sticking to a vegetarian or vegan diet, eating fermented foods alone is not enough. Make sure that you invest in a high-quality probiotic supplement as well.

Chapter 9

Fatty Acids:
The ABCs of Good Health

You may have already heard of the omega-3 fatty acids EPA (eicosapentaenoic acid) and DHA (docosahexaenoic acid) because of the key roles they play in cardiovascular, eye, brain, and emotional health (more on this later). These vital omega-3s are difficult to get from plant foods alone; the only direct sources are fish and fish oil supplements.

If you opt for a vegetarian or vegan diet, you must eat foods high in another omega-3, ALA (alpha-linolenic acid), as your body can convert ALA into EPA and DHA. These foods include:

Flaxseeds
Chia seeds
Walnuts
Fermented soybeans
Hemp seeds

There is one issue. The conversion rate is low. Only between 8 and 20 percent of ALA is converted to EPA, and between 0.5 and 9 percent of ALA is converted to DHA.[1] With such a low conversion rate, it's important to optimize it by making the following healthy changes to your diet:

- Eliminate foods cooked with trans-fatty acids—primarily fast foods and processed foods.
- Do not cook with sunflower, safflower, corn, cottonseed, and soybean oils. These are omega-6 oils and can decrease conversion by 40 percent.
- Decrease consumption of alcoholic beverages.

Regardless of whether you're a vegan or flexitarian, these changes can benefit your health enormously.

There's another omega-3 fatty acid that can help: SDA (stearidonic acid). The body converts SDA to EPA, but at a higher rate than the ALA. The best source of SDA is hemp seeds,[2] especially hemp seed oil. Hemp seed oil is also a rich source of ALA.[3] (See Chapter 3 for more on hemp seeds.)

Essential for Good Health

As mentioned earlier, the omegas are essential for good health. Omega-3 DHA and EPA are best known for their heart health benefits.[4] They help lower LDL (the "bad" cholesterol), triglycerides, and blood pressure. And they increase HDL (the "good" cholesterol).[5]

DHA and EPA are also crucial for brain and emotional health, and are key for proper brain development in children of all ages. Research has shown that DHA is a part of every brain cell[6] and both DHA and EPA can slow down the brain's aging.[7]

Good eye health, too, depends on getting enough DHA and EPA, as the retina has one of the highest concentrations of omega-3 fatty acids. One study showed that participants with the highest intake of EPA and DHA were 30 percent less likely to develop diseases of the retina compared to those participants with the lowest intake.[8] Another study demonstrated that with only a 2 percent increase, there was approximately a 40 to 50 percent decrease in the severity of retinopathy, a disease of the retina.[9]

The Omega 6 family of fatty acids is important, too. Omega 6s stimulate skin and hair growth, maintain bone health and the reproductive system, regulate metabolism, and are important for healthy brain functions.[10] Great sources include nuts and seeds, which are also sources of omega-3s.

Gamma-linolenic acid (GLA), one type of omega-6, stimulates fat burning and raises your metabolism.[11] It's also used to treat many health issues, including skin conditions, rheumatoid arthritis, and premenstrual syndrome (PMS). The best sources are evening primrose oil, borage oil, and black currant seed oil.

Both omega-3 and omega-6 fatty acids are known for their anti-inflammatory properties. Chronic inflammation is now considered the main cause of many serious illnesses, including heart disease, cancer, and Alzheimer's disease. But balance is key. For omega-6 and omega-3 to be the most effective, they have to be in balance with one another. The ideal ratio, according to many experts, is one-to-one or two-to-one, omega-6 to omega-3. In addition to getting all the benefits previously discussed, a good ratio also optimizes your ability to burn fat.[12]

Unfortunately, the ratio of omega-6s to omega-3s in the typical American diet is 15-to-1. That's primarily the result of eating processed and fast foods that are loaded with soybean, canola, and vegetable oils, all of which are high in omega-6 fatty acids.

Part 4

Lifestyle: It Matters

Health is a state of complete harmony of the body, mind, and spirit."

—B.K.S. Iyengar

Lifestyle Matters

Health is not just about your diet. Your lifestyle—including your career/work, social life, spiritual practice, and relationships—also affects your health. Some aspects of your lifestyle have more of a direct impact on your health and weight loss, and those are the ones that are covered in this section.

Chapter 10

Channel Your Inner Sleeping Beauty

Never underestimate the power of getting enough sleep every night. Sleeping well makes you more energetic, happy, and clearheaded, and it can help you manage, or even lose, weight.

When you suffer from sleep deprivation, three important hormones—leptin, ghrelin, and cortisol—become imbalanced and create a disconnect between your brain and stomach.

The body produces less leptin,[1] a hormone that tells the brain, "I'm full. Stop eating." A study published in 2004 shows that people with a 20 percent drop in leptin had a 24 percent increase in hunger and appetite. That drove them to eat high-calorie, salty snacks and high-carbohydrate foods, especially those that are sweet and starchy.[2]

While sleep deprivation causes leptin production to *decrease*, it causes an *increase* in the hormone ghrelin. Ghrelin, also known as the "hunger hormone," is secreted by the stomach when it's empty and sends a message to your brain that you're hungry.[3] Sleep studies show that ghrelin levels soar from lack of sleep, triggering a huge appetite and cravings for high-carb foods.

Like ghrelin, if you don't get enough sleep, the body produces too much of the hormone cortisol,[4] which also sends the signal that you're hungry. Studies have shown that cortisol doesn't just increase hunger, but it also increases consumption of comfort foods, like chocolate cake.[5]

With too little ghrelin, and too much leptin and cortisol, you overeat throughout the day without ever getting the sensation and satisfaction that you've had enough. As you can imagine, over time this can cause a significant amount of weight gain.

To help you get more sleep, try some of the following:

- Turn off all electronics, including your Wi-Fi system, at bedtime.
- Use an acupressure mat.
- Drink chamomile or valerian root tea at bedtime.
- Cut back or eliminate caffeine. Never have it after 3:00 p.m.
- Incorporate more cardiovascular exercise into your daily routine. Try walking more and taking the stairs instead of the elevator.
- Go to bed and wake up at the same time every day.
- Reduce stress (see Chapter 11).
- Do yoga asanas (poses) and meditate.

Chapter 11

Tame the Stress Monster

Chronic stress can do as much damage to your health and well-being as a terrible diet. It can cause you to gain weight and visceral fat[1,2] and can interfere with getting a good night's sleep. Stress depletes your brain's serotonin supply. And, like sleep deprivation, it causes too much cortisol, which increases blood sugar and insulin.

In a sense, cortisol is just doing its job. Its function is to increase blood sugar to give you an energy boost when you're in danger—e.g., you hear someone breaking into your home. The problem is, cortisol is also produced to deal with other types of stressful situations, like a bad job or relationship. Until you get these stressors under control, your body will continue to pump out more cortisol to help you cope.

As discussed in Chapter 10, the problem with too much cortisol is it makes you overeat and creates visceral fat. Cortisol sends a signal to your brain that you're hungry, and makes you reach for comfort foods that are high in fat and sugar.[3]

Chronic stress also affects your emotional health and wellness. During prolonged periods of stress, your body's supply of serotonin—a natural antidepressant and mood regulator—is used up to try to keep you calm and centered.[4] Serotonin is also needed to help you sleep well. Sleep deprivation creates hormone imbalances that cause weight gain and other health issues. Your body reacts to the serotonin deficiency (and sleep deprivation) by creating cravings for sweets and refined carbohydrates—our comfort foods.[5]

To increase serotonin, get some sun and supplement with Rhodiola and 5-HTP (see Chapter 6). Until you get control of the stressful situations in your life, there's another adaptogenic herb that can help: Ashwagandha. Ashwagandha has been shown in studies to reduce cortisol levels by up to 30 percent.

Other ways to reduce stress include:

- Acupuncture
- An acupressure mat
- Adequate sleep (eight hours every night)
- Eliminating caffeine, sugar, and alcohol
- Listening to recorded sounds of nature
- Yoga asanas
- Meditation
- Deep-breathing exercises (yoga pranayama)
- Movement/exercise
- Aromatherapy—specifically, lavender
- Essential oils

Chapter 12

Cook Like Your Great-Grandmother

Your great-grandmother, or possibly your grandmother, did not have access to processed and fast foods, as very few existed. They cooked what was available, which was proteins from animals raised on traditional farms, and whole, locally grown fruits and vegetables.

If you cook the same way, you can eliminate the added sugars and unhealthy grains and fats from your diet relatively quickly to improve your health and accelerate weight loss.

That can be difficult at first, as processed foods are convenient, cheap, and engineered to taste great. Let's face it, processed and fast foods have simplified our lives. Plus, with 600,000 processed food items[1] to choose from, we're not likely to get bored anytime soon.

> Ninety percent of the food in mainstream stores is processed, and only 10 percent is fresh, whole foods. The reverse was true during your grandmother's or great-grandmother's time.

Processed foods may fit our modern, busy lifestyles, but the majority are laden with chemicals and artificial colors and flavors, many of which are linked to illnesses.[2] What's more, most have no nutrition to speak of, are engineered to keep you eating, and contain lots of sugar, salt, unhealthy fats, and soy by-products.

Overweight, Overfed, and Undernourished

Processed foods contain minuscule amounts of vitamins, minerals, and other needed nutrients, like phytonutrients and antioxidants. To get the nutrition our bodies need, we instinctively keep eating, which has created a large population of people in the U.S. who are overfed, overweight, and undernourished.

The fiber is also missing, which is another reason why processed foods make us fat. The fiber is removed to extend the product's shelf life.[3] It allows the food to cook faster, to be frozen without changing its texture and mouthfeel, and to be shipped globally.[4] But fiber is needed to slow down digestion and the absorption of sugar into the bloodstream. It gets you full faster, keeps you full longer, and helps keep your blood sugar balanced so that less sugar is converted to fat.

Engineered to Get You Hooked

Food companies spend a lot of time and money to engineer their products to taste great, stimulate your appetite, and get you hooked. Salt, fat, and sugar do just that, and it's precisely why all three are used in 80 percent of processed foods. Added sugar, in particular, is incredibly addictive.

Are Loaded with HFCS and Added Sugar

As we discussed, processed foods are loaded with high-fructose corn syrup (HFCS) and refined, added sugar. These unhealthy ingredients are linked to serious illnesses, premature aging, and obesity (see Chapter 5).

Contain Unhealthy, Soy By-Products

Soy by-products are in 60 percent of all processed and packaged foods, and close to 100 percent of fast foods.[5] This is mainly due to the U.S. government's Farm Bill that provides massive subsidies to farms that grow soy. Between 1995 and 2014, soy subsidies totaled $31.8 billion.[6] While some of the soy is used to feed livestock, the rest gets added to processed foods.

Based on those numbers, you would think that these by-products are safe. They absolutely are not. Soy by-products are created using questionable, unhealthy processes, and, like all unfermented soy products, they can lead to health issues (see Chapter 3).

You'll find different names and types of soy by-products listed on food labels as follows:

- Soy protein isolate (SPI)
- Textured vegetable protein (TVP) (Most are made from soy.)
- Textured plant protein
- Soy protein concentrates
- Hydrolyzed vegetable protein
- Mono-diglyceride

- Soya, soja, or yuba
- Lecithin (Although it's sometimes made from other sources, like eggs or sunflower.)
- MSG (monosodium glutamate)

Always read labels carefully to see what the product contains. When you do, you'll be more inclined to stop consuming these products. Nothing can beat a diet that consists of whole, fresh foods for your health and well-being.

A Processed Food Is Still a Processed Food

Many processed-food companies are jumping on the "healthy" bandwagon. To add new marketing claims[7] and to penetrate specialty markets, like those discussed below, it's simple to do a re-engineering and repackaging of existing products.

Gluten-free, fat-free, low-fat, all natural, vegetarian, and vegan are hot niche markets for food companies. But are these products any healthier than other processed foods? The answer is, it depends. Fat-free and low-fat foods are high in sugar. Fat is flavorful, so when you remove it, you remove the flavor as well. To add flavor back in, sugar—and a lot of it—is added. These are definitely not healthy products. We need to eliminate added sugar and get *more* healthy fats into our diet instead.

The popular "all natural" label is sorely misleading. Most people believe it means the food does not contain harmful additives, ingredients, or anything artificial. Not true. The Food and Drug Administration (FDA) has not yet devised a formal definition. Currently, it considers the word "natural" to mean nothing artificial or synthetic was added *"that would normally be expected to be in that food.*[8]*"* This is an incredibly vague statement that can mean just about anything.

Another label frequently used is "natural flavors." Unfortunately, this still allows unhealthy ingredients to be added. For example, a product can contain up to 20 percent of MSG, a chemical flavor enhancer, and still use that label.[9]

Food companies use rice flour, tapioca starch, potato flour, and other gluten-free grains to make gluten-free products. These flours may be gluten-free, but they have a lot of starch. As you know by now, a high starch food will spike your blood sugar, cause you to gain weight, and possibly cause other health issues.

Substitutes like quinoa flour are better than other gluten-free flours, but they usually mix it with a cheaper, high-starch flour, like rice. For example, I've noticed a "made with quinoa" claim on the front packaging of pasta products, but there is no mention of the rice flour. You'll think it's 100 percent quinoa unless you read the back label. That can be grossly misleading to the unwary consumer.

Also misleading is the perception that a food labeled vegetarian or vegan is healthy. Some brands use the same unhealthy ingredients found in other processed foods, including unhealthy fats, added sugars, wheat and wheat gluten, and many of the soy by-products listed above.

Mock meats can be the biggest offenders. They're super convenient and come in the form of hot dogs, hamburgers, chicken wings, barbecue beef, etc. Plus, they're easy to find; they're now available in most conventional grocery stores. Unfortunately, most mock meats contain soy by-products, wheat gluten, and high amounts of sodium, preservatives, and hydrogenated fats. And, because of their convenience, they have now become a mainstay of vegetarian and vegan diets.

You can find healthier mock meats made with beans, mushrooms, and grains, particularly the mock hamburgers. These may help you during your transition to a vegetarian or vegan diet and are good in a pinch when you don't have time to cook. They certainly are better than grabbing a pizza or other fast food, but don't become reliant on them; they still lack the nutritional value you get from whole, unprocessed foods.

Chapter 13

Crank Up Your Metabolism

To burn more calories instead of storing them as fat, it's important to optimize your metabolism. You can do this in many ways—e.g., build more muscle, do cardiovascular exercise, get enough protein, and eat the right fats.

Build Muscle

Our bodies are always burning calories, even when we're not moving. That's called the resting metabolic rate, and it's based on muscle mass. Every pound of muscle uses approximately six calories daily to sustain itself, so the more muscle you have, the higher the rate. Muscles play another role in weight loss: When they're active, they burn fat for fuel.[1]

Move

It may not come as a surprise to you that aerobic exercise burns calories, but did you know that high-intensity, aerobic exercise can keep your metabolism higher *hours after* your workout? According to some studies, it does, although no one knows why.[2] What we do know is, the body starts using more fat and fewer carbohydrates after a hard workout.[3]

Exercise also produces HGH (human growth hormone). HGH is a hormone needed for many functions, including muscle growth and repair, and sugar and fat metabolism. Our bodies make less HGH as we age. Less HGH causes more body fat and less muscle mass, which slows our resting metabolism and ability to burn fat.

Eat Foods That Boost Metabolism

Getting enough protein, and the right fats and fatty acids into your diet can also increase your metabolism.

GLA (gamma-linolenic acid) is an omega-6 fatty acid that has been shown to be effective for weight loss as it stimulates the thyroid gland to raise the body's metabolism.[4] The best sources are evening primrose oil, borage oil, and black currant seed oil supplements.

Omega-3 essential fatty acids help optimize your body's ability to burn body fat for fuel. Plant foods high in omega-3s include flaxseeds, hemp seeds, and chia seeds (see Chapter 4).

Protein also plays a role in metabolism and weight loss. It optimizes HGH levels, which, as stated earlier, are essential for muscle growth and repair. The more lean muscles you have, the higher your resting metabolism, which means your body will burn more calories when you're inactive.

Oils that contain medium-chain fats (MCFs), including coconut oil, can also raise your metabolism. They increase stamina and your body's ability to burn fat.

> *"Vegetarians have been observed to have a slightly higher rate of metabolism during rest, meaning they burn up slightly more of their ingested calories as body heat rather than depositing them as body fat."*—The China Study

Chapter 14

Keep Moving

Throughout this book, we talked about exercise, particularly cardiovascular, and how it's essential to a healthy lifestyle and for weight loss. I think
it's worth repeating those benefits here and adding
others that haven't been mentioned.

- Boosts your metabolism
- Burns calories instead of storing them as fat
- Burns stored fat[1]
- Burns off liver fat[2]
- Is needed for a healthy cardiovascular sys-
  tem
- Lowers blood pressure
- Reduces cortisol levels
- Helps you sleep
- Influences new brain-cell growth[3]

- Helps build new networks in the brain[4]
- Makes brain neurons nimble and able to multitask[5]
- Is a potent anti-inflammatory[6]
- Boosts moods
- Lowers stress

If you're relatively sedentary, start slow and always with something you enjoy. Most people find it easier to begin by building exercise into their everyday routine. For example, if possible, walk to work or the store instead of jumping in the car. Take the stairs instead of the elevator. Or simply walk briskly every day for 15 to 20 minutes. Once this becomes easy, start experimenting to find out what other forms of exercise you enjoy and add it to your routine.

It's no longer necessary to get to a gym to take an exercise or yoga class. There are lots of classes that you can stream online, and most do not require equipment (see Chapter 15). This saves lots of time getting to and from the gym. And, classes range from 15 minutes to an hour, so you can always fit something into your schedule.

Remember that routines get boring, and boredom can cause you to give up your exercise routine. So, when you're bored or no longer inspired, mix it up by trying something new. Another useful technique to keep you on track is to team up with someone. Research shows that having a workout partner is key to getting more exercise.[7]

Always check with your doctor before beginning any strenuous exercise program.

Part 5

Where to Begin

"Start by doing what is necessary, then do what is possible, and suddenly you are doing the impossible."

—St. Francis of Assisi (1182–1226)

Chapter 15

Tips for Transitioning

Everyone is different, so no one can tell you which plant-based diet is right for you or the best way to make the changes discussed in this book. But there are some things you can do that are helpful to anyone transitioning.

Don't Rush It

Start slowly if your goal is to go vegetarian or vegan. According to an independent study conducted by the research group Faunalytics, people that transition quickly to a vegetarian or vegan diet are less likely to stick with it.[1] Instead, consider starting, for example, by eliminating animal protein from just one or two of your daily meals. Or you can eliminate it only on specific days of the week. Another option is to start by giving up one type of animal protein, perhaps red meat. As you adjust to the change, you can then eliminate poultry or fish. If your goal is a vegan diet, once you've adjusted to not eating meat, you can then focus on eliminating dairy and other animal products, like cheese.

At some point during the elimination process, you may decide that a flexitarian diet is better for you. A flexitarian diet is a healthy choice as long as you consume only grass-fed beef; free-range, organic poultry; and wild-caught fish that has the least amount of mercury, like sardines and salmon.

Regardless of how you start, don't focus solely on giving up meat. Crowd the animal protein out of your diet by adding lots of whole foods, including healthy nuts, seeds, fruits, and vegetables. But take this slowly as well. Your digestive track needs to get accustomed to all the added fiber; initially, a lot of fiber or raw vegetables can cause gas, bloating, and cramps.

In addition to transitioning to a plant-based diet, there are other recommendations in this book that will optimize your health and lead to sustainable weight loss. Do not try to incorporate all of these changes into your diet all at once. Pick one change, achieve it, and only then add another change to your diet. I think one of the best places to start is by eliminating processed or fast foods. It may take some time to achieve this goal, as you need to adjust to spending more time shopping and preparing meals. But the upside is, you tackle several issues all at once; you minimize a lot of added sugars, unhealthy fats, and grains, and get a lot more nutrition and fiber into your diet.

Plan Out Your Meals

Plan out your meals for the entire week. The most common reasons people give for eating meat again are constant hunger, lack of energy, and boredom, which can all be avoided by some simple planning.

Planning makes it easier to get the nutrition, protein, and fat you need to feel satisfied throughout each day. It also keeps you from getting into bad habits, like eating fast and processed foods instead of healthy whole foods. When you plan ahead, it's also easier to keep things interesting instead of falling into a rut and eating the same thing all the time.

Cook Once and Eat Twice

To save lots of time, always cook enough for two meals. You can freeze a portion for another meal or take it to work the next day for lunch. Of course, not all recipes lend themselves well to freezing or travel, but I find that many do.

Keep It Simple

Unless you have a lot of spare time on your hands and you're an experienced cook, don't start your new diet with elaborate recipes. Complicated recipes and advanced cooking techniques will just frustrate you, and you'll be back to your old diet in no time.

Some recipes are easy to convert to vegetarian or vegan dishes. Take chili, for example: Just replace the ground meat with black beans, pinto beans, or a combination of both. Think about recipes that you already cook that can easily be transformed, like burritos.

Soups and salads are also a great help during the early transition stage. Simple vegetarian soups and hardy salads are easy to put together and can provide you with the protein, fat, and carbohydrates that you need for a balanced meal. For example, to get enough protein into a salad, add cold chickpeas and walnuts or hard-boiled eggs.

Be a Restaurant Detective

Don't despair. You don't have to eat in a vegetarian or vegan restaurant. Many restaurants will let you select several side dishes in place of one of their entrées. There are also ethnic restaurants that have a big selection of vegetarian entrées, like Italian, Chinese, Mexican, Indian, Japanese, Spanish, and Thai. These are excellent choices when dining out with friends and family that are carnivores.

But, before deciding, check them out online. Most restaurants post their menus. If they don't, call ahead and check to see if they can accommodate you.

Pack Some On-the-Go Quality Foods

When you know you'll be away from home all day, bring healthy snacks, like fresh fruit or nuts and dried fruit. Liquid protein shakes are also great to take with you. Some brands are available in an individual serving size. They're easy to grab on the way out the door and will keep you satiated while you're out and about throughout the day.

When you go on vacation, it's extremely helpful to pack a high-quality, vegetarian protein powder or powdered meal replacement to ensure that you get the necessary nutrition and protein while you're away. You'll spend less time worrying about food and more time enjoying your vacation.

Chapter 16

Helpful Resources for Your Transition and Beyond

I've listed below some resources and products that I'm confident you'll find useful during and beyond your transition:

Food Directories

Natural food stores and health food stores.
www.greenpeople.org/healthfood.html

All-natural, organic food directory.
www.organicstorelocator.com/

List of farmers' markets and food coops throughout

the USA.
http://www.localharvest.org/farmers-markets/

Vegetarian and vegan guide to restaurants.
www.happycow.net/

Eat Well Guide Online.
Directory of local, sustainable foods, including family farms, markets, restaurants, and more.
www.eatwellguide.org

Food Resources

Produce Made Simple.
Just about everything you need to know about produce, including what goes well with what, how to select and store, how to prepare, nutrient content, recipes, different varieties, and lots more.
producemadesimple.ca/

CROM-O-Meter.
Free resources to track your nutrition, fitness, and health data.
https://cronometer.com/

United States Department of Agriculture, Food Composition Database.

Search this database to find the nutrient information for your food items. Also lets you generate
lists of foods sorted by nutrient content.
https://ndb.nal.usda.gov/ndb/

SELF Nutrition Database.
Detailed online nutrition information and analysis
tools.
http://nutritiondata.self.com/

Kitchen Tools

I don't believe that you need a lot of fancy
kitchen appliances to make good food. But you'll
find a high-speed blender invaluable for getting
more fruits and vegetables into your diet and for
making your food more exciting.

There are several high-speed blenders available, but these two are the ones that I have used
and am happy with:

Vitamix
https://www.vitamix.com/home

NutriBullet
https://nutribullet.com/

Cookbooks

There are too many good cookbooks to list, but *How to Cook Everything Vegetarian* by Mark Bittman is not just recipes. It also teaches you everything you need to know about cooking in general—terrific for novices.

If you're athletic and plan to transition to a vegetarian or vegan diet, *Thrive Energy Cookbook: 150 Plant-Based Whole Food Recipes* by Brendan Brazier is a good choice.

Herbs and Supplement Directories

National Institute of Health: Herbs at a Glance.
A series of brief fact sheets that provide basic information about specific herbs or botanicals, including common names, the science, potential side effects and cautions, and additional resources.
https://nccih.nih.gov/health/herbsataglance.htm

MedlinePlus: Herbs and Supplements.
This directory provides information on the effectiveness, correct dosage, and potential drug interactions.
https://medlineplus.gov/druginformation.html

Stream Your Workouts and Yoga Classes

Stream online workouts from the comfort of your home.
www.DailyBurn.com

Fifty free workout resources online.
http://makeyourbodywork.com/how-to-exercise-at-home/

Stream or download asana and guided meditation classes.
https://www.gaia.com/

Recommended Reading

The books listed below are just some of the invaluable sources of information that I used for this book. They represent some of my favorite reads as well. You can find others in the reference section.

Eating on the Wild Side: The Missing Link to Optimum Health by Jo Robinson

The Diet Cure: The 8-Step Program to Rebalance Your Body Chemistry and End Food Cravings,

Weight Gain, and Mood Swings Naturally by Julia Ross, M.A.

Wheat Belly Total Health by William Davis, M.D.

The Blood Sugar Solution: The Ultrahealthy Program for Losing Weight, Preventing Disease, and Feeling Great Now! by Mark Hyman M.D.

Primal Bodies, Primal Minds: Beyond the Paleo Diet for Total Health and a Longer Life by Nora T. Gedgaudas, CNS, CNT

Fat Chance: Beating the Odds Against Sugar, Processed Food, Obesity, and Disease by Robert H. Lustig, M.D.

Your Miracle Brain by Jean Carper

Grain Brain: The Surprising Truth about Wheat, Carbs, and Sugar--Your Brain's Silent Killers by David Perlmutter, M.D.

The Healing Nutrients Within by Eric R. Braverman, M.D.

Notes

Part 1: Why a Plant-Based Diet

Chapter 2: The Undeniable Benefits

1. Campbell, T.C., Stone, G. (2011). Forks Over Knives: The Plant-Based Way to Health. New York, NY: The Experiment, LLC.

2. Snowdon D A. Animal product consumption and mortality because of all causes combined, coronary heart disease, stroke, diabetes, and cancer in Seventh-day Adventists. *Am J Clin Nutr*. 1988; 48 (3 Suppl):739-48.

3. Key TJ, Fraser GE, Thorogood M, Appleby PN, Beral V, Reeves G. Mortality in vegetarians and nonvegetarians: detailed findings from a collaborative analysis of 5 prospective studies. *Am J Clin Nutr*. 1999; 70, 516S-524S.

4. Rouse IL, Armstrong BK, Beilin LJ, Vandongen R. Blood-pressure-lowering effect of a vegetarian diet: controlled trial in normotensive subjects. *Lancet*. 1983;1:5-10.

5. Rouse IL, Belin LJ, Mahoney DP, et al. Nutrient intake, blood pressure, serum and urinary prostaglandins and serum thromboxane B2 in a controlled trial with a lacto-ovo-vegetarian diet. *J Hypertension*. 1986;4:241-50.

6. Margetts BM, Beilin LJ, Armstrong BK, Vandongen R. A randomized controlled trial of a vegetarian diet in the treatment of mild hypertension. *Clin Exp Pharmacol Physiol*. 1985 May-Jun;12(3):263-6.

7. Margetts BM, Beilin LJ, Vandongen R, Armstrong BK. Vegetarian diet in mild hypertension: a randomised controlled trial. *Br Med J*. 1986 Dec 6; 293(6560): 1468–1471.

8. Lindahl O, Lindwall L, Spangberg A, Stenram A, Ockerman PA. A vegan regimen with reduced medication in the treatment of hypertension. *Br J Nutr*. 1984;52:11-20.

9. West RO, Hayes OB. Diet and serum cholesterol levels: a comparison between vegetarians and nonvegetarians in a Seventh-day Adventist group. *Am J Clin Nutr*. 1968;21:853-62.

10. Sacks FM, Ornish D, Rosner B, McLanahan S, Castelli WP, Kass EH. Plasma lipoprotein levels in vegetarians: the effect of ingestion of fats from dairy products. *JAMA*. 1985;254:1337-41.

11. Fisher M, Levine PH, Weiner B, et al. The effect of vegetarian diets on plasma lipid and platelet levels. *Arch Inter Med*. 1986;146:1193-7.

12. Burslem J, Schonfeld G, Howald M, Weidman SW, Miller JP. Plasma apoprotein and lipoprotein lipid levels in vegetarians. *Metabolism*. 1978;27:711-9.

13. Braverman, E. R. (1987). The Healing Nutrients Within (3rd ed.). Laguna Beach, CA: Basic Health Publications, Inc.

14. Physicians Committee for Responsible Medicine. Vegetarian Diets: Advantages for Children.

15 Block G. Epidemiologic evidence regarding vitamin C and cancer. *Am J Clin Nutr.* 1991;54:1310S-4S.

16. Craig WJ. Phytochemicals: guardians of health. *J Am Diet Assoc.* 1997,97(Suppl 2): S199-S204.

17. Braverman, E. R. (1987). The Healing Nutrients Within (3rd ed.). Laguna Beach, CA: Basic Health Publications, Inc.

18. Stone, G. (2011). Forks Over Knives: The Plant-Based Way to Health. New York, NY: The Experiment, LLC.

19. Beezhold, BL, Johnston, CS. Restriction of meat, fish, and poultry in omnivores improves mood: A pilot randomized controlled trial. *Nutrition Journal.* 14 February 2012

20. Appleby PN, Thorogood M, Mann J, Key TJ. Low body mass index in non-meat eaters: the possible roles of animal fat, dietary fibre and alcohol. *Int J Obes Relat Metab Disord.* 1998; 22: 454–460.

21. Newby PK, Katherine LT, Wolk A. Risk of overweight and obesity among semivegetarian, lactovegetarian, and vegan women. *Am J Clin Nutr.* 2005; 81: 1267–1274.

22. Spencer EA, Appleby PN, Davey GK, Key TJ. Diet and body mass index in 38000 EPIC-Oxford meat-eaters, fish-eaters, vegetarians and vegans. *Int J Obes Relat Metab Disord.* 2003; 27: 728–734.

23. Key T, Davey G. Prevalence of obesity is low in people who do not eat meat. *Br Med J* 1996; 313: 816–817.

24. They Eat What? What are They Feeding Animals on Factory Farms? Organic Consumers Association https://www.organicconsumers.org/news/they-eat-what-what-are-they-feeding-animals-factory-farms

25. Michael Greger, M.D. "Why is Meat a Risk Factor for Diabetes" Aug. 21, 2015

26. Uribarri J, Woodruff S, Goodman S, Cai W, Chen X, Pyzik R, Yong A, Striker G, Vlassara H. Advanced Glycation End Products in Foods and a Practical Guide to Their Reduction in the Diet. *J Am Diet Assoc.* 2010 June; 110(6): 911–16.e12. doi:10.1016/j.jada.2010.03.018.

27. Lichtenstein AH, Appel LJ, Brands M, Carnethon M, Daniels S, Franch HA, Franklin B, Kris- Etherton P, Harris WS, Howard B, Karanja N, Lefevre M, Rudel L, Sacks F, Van Horn L, Winston M, Wylie-Rosett J. Diet and lifestyle recommendations revision 2006: A scientific statement from the American Heart Association Nutrition Committee. Circulation. 2006; 114:82–96. [PubMed: 16785338]

28. World Cancer Research Fund/American Institute for Cancer Research. Food, Nutrition, Physical Activity, and the Prevention of Cancer: a Global Perspective. Washington, DC: American Institute for Cancer Research; 2007.

29. American Diabetes Association position statement: Nutrition recommendations and interventions for Diabetes. Diabetes Care. 2008; 31(Suppl):S61–S78. [PubMed: 18165339]

30. Uribarri J, Woodruff S, Goodman S, Cai W, Chen X, Pyzik

R, Yong A, Striker G, Vlassara H. Advanced Glycation End Products in Foods and a Practical Guide to Their Reduction in the Diet. *J Am Diet Assoc.* 2010 June; 110(6): 911–16.e12. doi:10.1016/j.jada.2010.03.018.

31. Segasothy M, Phillips PA. Vegetarian Diet: panacea for modern lifestyle diseases? *QJM*. 1999 Sep;92(9):531-44.

32. Stone, G. (2011). Forks Over Knives: The Plant-Based Way to Health. New York, NY: The Experiment, LLC.

33. The Minority Staff of the United States Senate Committee on Agriculture, Nutrition, and Forestry (Dec. 1997). Animal Waste Pollution in America: An Emerging National Problem.

34. Bland, A. "Is the Livestock Industry Destroying the Planet? For the earth's sake, maybe it's time we take a good, hard look at our dietary habits," Smithsonian.com. Aug. 1, 2012

35. Stone, G. (2011). Forks Over Knives: The Plant-Based Way to Health. New York, NY: The Experiment, LLC.

36. FAONewsroom. Food and Agriculture Organization of the United Nations."Livestock a major threat to environment. Remedies urgently needed." Nov. 29, 2006

Part 2: Macronutrients

Chapter 3: Protein: Much Ado About Everything

1. Gedgaudas, N. T. (2009). Primal Bodies, Primal Minds: Beyond the Paleo Diet for Total Health and a Longer Life. Rochester, VT: Healing Arts Press

2. University Maryland Medical Center Website. "Protein in

Diet," "Protein"

3. Johnston CS, Tjonn SL, Swan PD. High-Protein, Low-Fat Diets Are Effective for Weight Loss and Favorably Alter Biomarkers in Healthy Adults, *JN the Journal of Nutrition*, 134:586-591, March 2004

4. Ibid.

5. Cooper RK, Cooper LL (2007). Flip the Switch, Lose the Weight: Proven Strategies to Fuel Your Metabolism and Burn Fat. New York, NY: Rodale, Inc.

6. Johnston CS, Tjonn SL, Swan PD. High-Protein, Low-Fat Diets Are Effective for Weight Loss and Favorably Alter Biomarkers in Healthy Adults, *JN the Journal of Nutrition*, 134:586-591, March 2004

7. Lustig, R. H. (2013). Fat Chance: Beating the Odds Against Sugar, Processed Food, Obesity, and Disease. New York, NY: Penguin Group.

8. USDA National Nutrient Database for Standard Reference, Release 23

9. Tarnopolsky MA, Atkinson SA, MacDougall JD, Chesley A, Phillips S, Schwarcz HP. Evaluation of protein requirements for trained strength athletes. *J Appl Physiol* (1985). 1992 Nov; 73(5):1986-95.

10. N.R. Rodriguez, N. M. DiMarco, and S. Langley. Nutrition and Athletic Performance. *Journal of the American Dietetic Association* 109, no. 3 (2009), 509-27)

11. USDA Food Composition Database

12. Braverman, E. R. (1987). The Healing Nutrients Within (3rd ed.). Laguna Beach, CA: Basic Health Publications, Inc.

13. Ibid.

14. Dr. David Williams. "Make these foods a bigger part of your diet to help lower cholesterol."

15. SELFNutritionData NutritionData.Self.com

16. Elaine Magee, MPH, RD, The Benefits of Flaxseed. Web-MD

17. The World's Healthiest Foods, Flaxseeds http://www.wh-foods.com/genpage.php?tname=foodspice&dbid=81

18. Donaldson MS. Nutrition and cancer: A review of the evidence for an anti-cancer diet. *Nutrition Journal*. Oct. 20, 2004, 20043:19

19. J.C. Callaway. Hempseed as a nutritional resource: An overview. Department of Pharmaceutical Chemistry, University of Kuopio, FIN-70211 Kuopio, Finland

20. SELFNutritionData nutritiondata.self.com

21. Ibid.

22. USDA Food Composition Databases

23. SELFNutritionData nutritiondata.self.com

24. Ibid.

25. Brazier, B. (2014). Thrive Energy Cookbook: 150 Plant-Based Whole Food Recipes. Boston, MA: Da Capo Press

26. USDA National Nutrient Database

27. USDA Food Composition Databases

28. Hyman, M. (2012). The Blood Sugar Solution: The Ultra-healthy Program for Losing Weight, Preventing Disease, and Feeling Great Now. New York, NY: Little, Brown and Company.

29. Pitchford, P. (1993). Healing with Whole Foods (3rd ed.). Berkeley, CA: North American Books.

30. Ibid.

31. Robinson, J. (2013). Eating on the Wild Side: The Missing Link to Optimum Health. New York, NY: Little, Brown and Company

32. Gedgaudas, N. T. (2009). Primal Bodies, Primal Minds: Beyond the Paleo Diet for Total Health and a Longer Life. Rochester, VT: Healing Arts Press

33. Weston A. Price Foundation. Soy Alert. http://www.westonaprice.org/soy-alert/

34. Ibid.

35. Ibid.

Other Resources

Environmental Working Group (EWG). The United States Farm

Subsidy Information http://farm.ewg.org/region.php?
fips=00000

Ornish, D. (1996). Dr. Dean Ornish's Program for Reversing
Heart Disease: The Only System Scientifically Proven to Re-
verse Heart Disease without Drugs or Surgery. New York, NY:
Random House, Inc.

Chapter 4: Fat: Your Unexpected Ally

1. Hyman, M (2016). Eat Fat, Get Thin. New York, NY: Little,
Brown and Company.

2. Lustig, R. H. (2013). Fat Chance: Beating the Odds Against
Sugar, Processed Food, Obesity, and Disease. New York, NY:
Penguin Group.

3. Ross, J. (2012). The Diet Cure: The 8-Step Program to
Rebalance Your Body Chemistry and End Food Cravings,
Weight Gain, and Mood Swings Naturally. New York, NY:
Penguin Group.

4. Ibid.

5. Hyman, M (2016). Eat Fat, Get Thin. New York, NY: Little,
Brown and Company.

6. Ross, J. (2012). The Diet Cure: The 8-Step Program to
Rebalance Your Body Chemistry and End Food Cravings,
Weight Gain, and Mood Swings Naturally. New York, NY:
Penguin Group.

7. Enig M, Fallon S (2006). Eat Fat, Lose Fat: The Healthy
Alternative to Trans Fats. New York, NY: Plume Books.

8. St-Onge MP, Bosarge A, Goree LL, Darnell B. Medium Chain Triglyceride Oil Consumption as Part of a Weight Loss Diet Does Not Lead to an Adverse Metabolic Profile When Compared to Olive Oil. *J Am Coll Nutr.* 2008 Oct;27(5): 547-52.

9. Astrup A, Dyerberg J, Elwood P, Hermansen K, Hu FB, Jakobsen MU, Kok, FJ, Krauss RM, Lecerf JM, LeGrand P, Nestel P, Risérus U, Sanders T, Sinclair A, Stender S, Tholstrup T, Willett WC. The Role of Reducing Intakes of Saturated Fat in the Prevention of Cardiovascular Disease: Where Does the Evidence Stand in 2010? *Am J. Clin. Nutr.* 93 (2011): 684-88

10. Ross, J. (2012). The Diet Cure: The 8-Step Program to Rebalance Your Body Chemistry and End Food Cravings, Weight Gain, and Mood Swings Naturally. New York, NY: Penguin Group

11. Gedgaudas, N. T. (2009). Primal Bodies, Primal Minds: Beyond the Paleo Diet for Total Health and a Longer Life. Rochester, VT: Healing Arts Press

Chapter 5: Carbohydrates: It's Complicated

1. Gedgaudas, N. T. (2009). Primal Bodies, Primal Minds: Beyond the Paleo Diet for Total Health and a Longer Life. Rochester, VT: Healing Arts Press

2. Ross, J. (2012). The Diet Cure: The 8-Step Program to Rebalance Your Body Chemistry and End Food Cravings, Weight Gain, and Mood Swings Naturally. New York, NY: Penguin Group.

3. Carper, G (2000). Your Miracle Brain. New York, NY: Harper Collins

4. Looking older: the effect of high blood sugar levels. Leiden University Medical Center. http://www.research.leiden.edu/news/looking-older-blood-sugar-plays-a-role.html

5. Carper, G (2000). Your Miracle Brain. New York, NY: Harper Collins

6. Robinson, J. (2013). Eating on the Wild Side: The Missing Link to Optimum Health. New York, NY: Little, Brown and Company

7. World's Healthiest Foods http://www.whfoods.com/genpage.php?tname=foodspice&dbid=128

8. Robinson, J. (2013). Eating on the Wild Side: The Missing Link to Optimum Health. New York, NY: Little, Brown and Company

9. Carbs and Cooking, Diabetes UK https://www.diabetes.org.uk/Guide-to-diabetes/Enjoy-food/Carbohydrates-and-diabetes/carbs-and-cooking/

10. Gedgaudas, N. T. (2009). Primal Bodies, Primal Minds: Beyond the Paleo Diet for Total Health and a Longer Life. Rochester, VT: Healing Arts Press

11. Davis, W. (2014). Wheat Belly, Total Health. New York, NY: Rodale, Inc.

12. Bohn T, Davidsson L, Walczyk T, Hurrell RF. Phytic Acid Added to White-Wheat Bread Inhibits Fractional Apparent Magnesium Absorption in Humans, The American Journal of Clinical Nutrition 79, no. 3 (March 2004); 418-23

13. Davis, W. (2015). Wheat Belly: 10-Day Grain Detox: Reprogram Your Body for Rapid Weight Loss and Amazing Health. New York, NY: Rodale, Inc.

14. Ramiel N. Living with Phytic Acid. Weston Price http://www.westonaprice.org/health-topics/living-with-phytic-acid/ March 26, 2010

15. Singh M and Krikorian D. Inhibition of trypsin activity in vitro by phytate. *J. Agric Food Chem., 30(4), pp 799-800* July 1982

16. Ramiel N. Living with Phytic Acid. Weston Price http://www.westonaprice.org/health-topics/living-with-phytic-acid/ March 26, 2010

17. Jonsson T et al. Agrarian Diet and Diseases of Affluence - Do Evolutionary Novel Dietary Lectins Cause Leptin Resistance? BMC Endocrine Disorders. Dec. 10, 2005

18. Ross, J. (2012). The Diet Cure: The 8-Step Program to Rebalance Your Body Chemistry and End Food Cravings, Weight Gain, and Mood Swings Naturally. New York, NY: Penguin Group.

19. Ibid.

20. Zioudrou C, Streaty RA, Klee WA. Opioid Peptides Derived from Food Proteins: The Exorphins. J *Biol Chem* 1979 Apr 10;254(7):2446-9.

21. Gedgaudas, N. T. (2009). Primal Bodies, Primal Minds: Beyond the Paleo Diet for Total Health and a Longer Life. Rochester, VT: Healing Arts Press

22. Ross, J. (2012). The Diet Cure: The 8-Step Program to Rebalance Your Body Chemistry and End Food Cravings, Weight Gain, and Mood Swings Naturally. New York, NY: Penguin Group.

23. Davis, W. (2015). Wheat Belly: 10-Day Grain Detox: Reprogram Your Body for Rapid Weight Loss and Amazing Health. New York, NY: Rodale, Inc.

24. Davis, W. (2014). Wheat Belly, Total Health. New York, NY: Rodale, Inc.

25. Foster-Powell, Holt SHA, Brand-Miller JC. Whole wheat bread increases blood sugar to a higher level than sucrose. International table of glycemic index and glycemic load values: 2002. *Am J Clin Nutr* 2002;76(1):5-56.

26. Ross, J. (2012). The Diet Cure: The 8-Step Program to Rebalance Your Body Chemistry and End Food Cravings, Weight Gain, and Mood Swings Naturally. New York, NY: Penguin Group.

27. Hyman, M. (2012). The Blood Sugar Solution: The Ultra-healthy Program for Losing Weight, Preventing Disease, and Feeling Great Now. New York, NY: Little, Brown and Company.

28. Ibid.

29. Ross, J. (2012). The Diet Cure: The 8-Step Program to Rebalance Your Body Chemistry and End Food Cravings, Weight Gain, and Mood Swings Naturally. New York, NY: Penguin Group.

30. Ibid.

31. Perlmutter, D. (2013). Grain Brain: The Surprising Truth about Wheat, Carbs, and Sugar--Your Brain's Silent Killers. New York, NY: Little, Brown and Company

32. Davis W. Is Your Thyroid Really Running the Show? http://www.wheatbellyblog.com/2016/08/thyroid-really-running-show/

33. Davis W. Muffin Top, Man Boobs, and Bagel Bumps. http://www.wheatbellyblog.com/2015/06/muffin-tops-man-boobs-and-bagel-bumps/

34. Roelfsema F, Pijl H, Keenan D.M., Veldhuis J.D. Prolactin Secretion in Healthy Adults is Determined by Gender, Age, and Body Mass Index. PLoS One. 2012; 7(2): e31305.

35. Fanciulli G, Dettori A, Demontis MP, Anania V, Delitala G. Serum Prolactin Levels after Administration of the Alimentary Opioid Peptide Gluten Exorphin B4 in Male Rats. *Nutritional Neuroscience*. 2004 Feb; 7(1): 53-5.

36. Johnson RE and Murad MH. Gynecomastia: Pathophysiology, Evaluation, and Management. Mayo Clinic Proceedings 2009 Nov; 84(11):1010-1015.

37. Lautenbach A, Budde A, Wrann CD, Teichmann B, Vieten G, Karl T, Nave H. Obesity and the Associated Mediators Leptin, Estrogen and IGF-I Enhance the Cell Proliferation and Early Tumorigenesis of Breast Cancer Cells. *Nutr Cancer*. 2009;61(4);484-91.

38. Key T, Appleby P, Barnes I, Reeves G; Endogenous Hormones and Breast Cancer Collaborative Group. Endogenous Sex Hormones and Breast Cancer in Postmenopausal Women:

Reanalysis of Nine Prospective Studies. *J Natl Cancer Inst.* 2002 Apr 17;94(8):606-16.

39. Ross, J. (2012). The Diet Cure: The 8-Step Program to Rebalance Your Body Chemistry and End Food Cravings, Weight Gain, and Mood Swings Naturally. New York, NY: Penguin Group.

40. Brazier, B. (2014). Thrive Energy Cookbook: 150 Plant-Based Whole Food Recipes. Boston, MA: Da Capo Press

41. Johnson RK, Appel LJ, Brands M, et al. Dietary sugars intake and cardiovascular health: a scientific statement from the American Heart Association. *Circulation* 2009 Sep 15;120(11):1011-20.

42. Harvard School of Public Health http://www.hsph.harvard.edu/nutritionsource/carbohydrates/added-sugar-in-the-diet/#ref27

43. Clays P, Deliens T, Huybrechts I, et al. Comparison of Nutritional Quality of the Vegan, Vegetarian, Semi-Vegetarian, Pesco-Vegetarian and Omnivorous Diet. *Nutrients.* 2014 Mar; 6(3): 1318–1332.

44. Lenoir M, Serre F, Cantin L, Ahmed SH (2007). Intense Sweetness Surpasses Cocaine Reward. *PLoS ONE* 2(8): e698.

45. Kessler D. (2009). The End of Overeating: Taking Control of the Insatiable American Appetite. New York, NY: Rodale, Inc.

46. DesMailsons K. (2008). Potatoes Not Prozac: Simple Solutions for Sugar Sensitivity New York: Simon & Schuster

47. Lenoir M, Serre F, Cantin L, Ahmed SH (2007). Intense Sweetness Surpasses Cocaine Reward. *PLoS ONE* 2(8): e698.

48. Stone, G. (2011). Forks Over Knives: The Plant-Based Way to Health. New York, NY: The Experiment, LLC.

49. Amo K, Aria H, Uebanso T, Fukaya M et al. Effects of xylitol on metabolic parameters and visceral fat accumulation. *J Clin Biochem Nutr.* 2011 Jul; 49(1): 1–7.

50. Ludwig DS. Artificially sweetened beverages: Cause for concern, *JAMA.* 2009 Dec 9;302(22): 2477-78

51. Swithers SE, Davidson TL. A role for sweet taste: calorie predictive relations in energy regulation by rats. *Behav Neurosci*, 2008; 122 (1): 161-73)

52. M.B Vos, Kimmons JE, Gillespie C, Welsh J, Blanck HM. Dietary Fructose Consumption among US Children and Adults: The Third National Health and Nutrition Examination Survey. *Medscape J. Med.* 2008 Jul 9;10(7):160.

53. Harvard Health Publications. Abundance of fructose not good for the liver, heart. http://www.health.harvard.edu/heart-health/abundance-of-fructose-not-good-for-the-liver-heart

54. Ibid.

55. Shapiro A, Wu W, Roncal C, Cheng KY, Johnson RJ, Scarpace PJ. Fructose-induced leptin resistance exacerbates weight gain in response to subsequent high-fat feeding. *Am J Physiol Regul Integr Comp Physiol* 2008 Nov;295(5):R1370-5

56. Parks EJ, Skokan LE, Timlin MT, Dingfelder CS. Dietary sugars stimulate fatty acid synthesis in adults. *J Nutr.* 2008

Jun;138(6):1039-46

57. W.I. Dillis. Protein Fructosylation: Fructose and the Maillard Reaction. *Am. J. Clin. Nutr.* 58 (1993): 779S-87S.

58. Lustig, R. H. (2013). Fat Chance: Beating the Odds Against Sugar, Processed Food, Obesity, and Disease. New York, NY: Penguin Group.

59. Davis, W. (2011). Wheat Belly: Lose the Wheat, Lose the Weight, and Find Your Path Back to Health. New York, NY: Rodale, Inc.

60. Bengmark S. Advanced glycation and lipoxidation end products - amplifiers of inflammation: The role of food. *JPEN J Parenter Enteral Nutr.* 2007 Sep-Oct;31(5):430-40.

61. Harvard Health Publications. Abundance of fructose not good for the liver, heart. http://www.health.harvard.edu/heart-health/abundance-of-fructose-not-good-for-the-liver-heart

62. Marcus, J. Glucose deprivation activates feedback loop that kills cancer cells, UCLA study shows, J June 26, 2012 UCLA Science + Technology http://newsroom.ucla.edu/releases/researchers-discover-that-glucose-235478

63. Graham NA, Tahmasian M, Kohli B, Komisopoulou E, Zhu M, Vivanco I, Teitell MA, Wu H, Ribas A, Lo RS, Ingo Mellinghoff K, Mischel PS, Graeber TG. Glucose deprivation activates a metabolic and signaling amplification loop leading to cell death. Mos Syst Biol. 2012, Jun 26;8:589.

64. University of Utah Health Sciences. Does Sugar Feed Cancer? August 18, 2009. ScienceDaily http://www.sciencedaily.com/releases/2009/08/090817184539.htm

65. Klement RJ and Kämmerer U. Is there a role for carbohydrate restriction in the treatment and prevention of cancer? *Nutr Metab* (Lond) 2011; 8: 75

66. Carper, G (2000). Your Miracle Brain. New York, NY: Harper Collins

67. Volta U, Tovoli F, Cicola R, Parisi C, Fabbri A, Piscaglia M, Fiorini E, Caio G. Serological Tests in Gluten Sensitivity (nonceliac Gluten Intolerance). *J Clin Gastroenterol* 2012 Sep; 46(8):680-5. doi: 10.1097/MCG.0b013e3182372541

68. S. Choi, Disilvio B, Fernstrom MH, Fernstrom JD. Meal Ingestion, Amino Acids, and Brain Neurotransmitters: Effects of Dietary Protein Source on Serotonin and Catecholamine Synthesis Rates. *Physiol Behav*. 2009 Aug 4;98(1-2):156-62

69. Lustig, R. H. (2013). Fat Chance: Beating the Odds Against Sugar, Processed Food, Obesity, and Disease. New York, NY: Penguin Group.

70. Carper, G (2000). Your Miracle Brain. New York, NY: Harper Collins

71. Ibid.

72. Ibid.

73. American Diabetes Association, Glycemic Index and Diabetes http://www.diabetes.org/food-and-fitness/food/what-can-i-eat/understanding-carbohydrates/glycemic-index-and-diabetes.html

74. Robinson, J. (2013). Eating on the Wild Side: The Missing Link to Optimum Health. New York, NY: Little, Brown and

Company

75. Mizoguchi T, Takehara I, Masuzawa T, Saito T, Naoki Y. Nutrigenomic studies of effects of Chlorella on subjects with high-risk factors for lifestyle-related disease. *J Med Food*. 2008 Sep;11(3):395-404

76. Atkins RC. (1998). Dr. Atkins' Vita-Nutrient Solution: Nature's Answer to Drugs. New York, NY: Simon & Schuster

77. Hyman, M. (2012). The Blood Sugar Solution: The Ultra-healthy Program for Losing Weight, Preventing Disease, and Feeling Great Now. New York, NY: Little, Brown and Company.

78. Carper, G (2000). Your Miracle Brain. New York, NY: Harper Collins

79. NIH National Institutes of Health. Chromium: What is it? https://ods.od.nih.gov/factsheets/Chromium-HealthProfessional/

80. Srivastava JK, Shankar E, Gupta S. Chamomile: A herbal medicine of the past with bright future. *Mol Med Rep*. 2010 Nov 1;3(6):895-901

81. Bijak M, Saluk J, Tsirigotis-Maniecka M, Komorowska H, Wachowicz et al. The influence of conjugates isolated from Matricaria chamomilla L. on platelets activity and cytotoxicity. *Int J Biol Macromol* 2013 Oct;61:218-29

Other Resources

Fed Up. Dir. Stephanie Soechtig. Atlas Films. 2014

Chapter 6: Withdrawal: The Biggest Hurdle

1. Avena NM, Rada P, Hoebel BG. Evidence for sugar addiction: Behavioral and neurochemical effects of intermittent, excessive sugar intake. *Neurosci Biobehav* Rev. 2008; 32(1): 20–39.

2. Davis, W. (2014). Wheat Belly, Total Health. New York, NY: Rodale, Inc.

3. Ibid.

4. Ibid.

5. Lishmanov IuB, Trifonova ZhV, Tsibin AN, Maslova LV, Dement'eva LA. Plasma beta-endorphin and stress hormones in stress and adaptation. *Biull Eksp Biol Med.* 1987 Apr;103(4): 422-4.

6. Davis, W. (2014). Wheat Belly, Total Health. New York, NY: Rodale, Inc.

7. Jukić T, Rojc B, Boben-Bardutzky D, Hafner D, Hafner M, Ihan A, The Use of a Food Supplementation with D-phenylalanine, L-Glutamine and L-5-Hydroxytriptophan in the Alleviation of Alcohol Withdrawal Symptoms. *Coll Antropol.* 2011 Dec;35(4):1225-30.

8. Hyman, M. (2014). The Blood Sugar Solution 10-Day Detox Diet: Activate Your Body's Natural Ability to Burn Fat and Lose Weight Fast. New York, NY: Little, Brown and Company

Part 3: Micronutrients

Chapter 7: Supplements: The Nonnegotiables

1. Ramiel N. Living with Phytic Acid. Weston Price http://www.westonaprice.org/health-topics/living-with-phytic-acid/ March 26, 2010

2. Choline, Linus Pauling Institute, Micronutrient Information Center, http://lpi.oregonstate.edu/mic/other-nutrients/choline

3. Ibid.

Chapter 8: Microflora: The Anti Antinutrient

1. Ramiel N. Living with Phytic Acid. Weston Price http://www.westonaprice.org/health-topics/living-with-phytic-acid/ March 26, 2010

2. Michael S. Donaldson, "Nutrition and cancer: A review of the evidence for an anti-cancer diet." *Nutrition Journal* 2004 3:19

3. Rachel Champeau | May 28, 2013. "Changing gut bacteria through diet affects brain function, UCLA study shows." http://newsroom.ucla.edu/releases/changing-gut-bacteria-through-245617

4. Famularo G, De Simone C, Pandey V, Sahu AR, Minisola G. Probiotic lactobacilli: an innovative tool to correct the malabsorption syndrome of vegetarians? *Med Hypotheses*. 2005;65(6):1132-5. Epub 2005 Aug 10.

Chapter 9: Fatty Acids: The ABCs of Good Health

1. Daniells, S. Omega-3: ALA intakes enough for EPA/DPA levels for non-fish eaters? NUTRA ingredients-usa.com. Nov 8, 2010.

2. Callaway J.C., Tennil T., Pate D.W. Occurrence of "omega-3" stearidonic acid (cis-6,9,12,15- octadecatetraenoic acid) in hemp (Cannabis sativa L.) seed. *Journal of the International Hemp Association* 1996 3(2): 61-63.

3. Ibid.

4. Swanson D, Block R, Mousa SA. Omega-3 Fatty Acids EPA and DHA: Health Benefits Throughout Life. *Adv Nutr.* 2012 Jan; 3(1): 1–7.

5. University of Maryland Medical Center. Data sheet. Omega-3 fatty acids

6. Ibid.

7. Omega-3 Supplements May Slow A Biological Effect of Aging, The Ohio State University, http:// researchnews.osu.edu/archive/omega3aging.htm

8. SanGiovanni JS, Agrón E, Meleth AD, Reed GF, Sperduto RD, Clemons TE, Chew EY. Long-chain polyunsaturated fatty acid intake and 12-y incidence of neovascular age-related macular degeneration and central geographic atrophy: AREDS report 30, a prospective cohort study from the Age-Related Eye Disease Study. *Am J Clin Nutr.* 2009 Dec; 90(6): 1601-1607.

9. NIH National Institute Health. Omega-3 Fatty Acids Protect

Eyes Against Retinopathy, Study Finds. June 24, 2007 http://www.nih.gov/news/pr/jun2007/nei-24.htm

10. University Maryland Medical Center. Omega-6 Fatty Acids. http://umm.edu/health/medical/altmed/supplement/omega6-fatty-acids

11. Ross, J. (2012). The Diet Cure: The 8-Step Program to Rebalance Your Body Chemistry and End Food Cravings, Weight Gain, and Mood Swings Naturally. New York, NY: Penguin Group.

12. Kuss T. (1992). A Guidebook to Clinical Nutrition for the Health Professional: General Uses and Proven Applications of the Systemic Formulas. Pleasant Hill, CA: Institute of Bioenergetic Research

Part 4: Lifestyle: It Matters

Chapter 10: Channel Your Inner Sleeping Beauty

1. S. Taheri, Lin L, Austin D, Young T, Mignot E. Short Sleep Duration Is Associated with Reduced Leptin, Elevated Ghrelin, and Increased Body Mass Index. *PLoS Med.* 2004 Dec;1(3):e62

2. Spiegel K, Tasali E, Penev P, Van Cauter E. Brief Communication: Sleep Curtailment in Healthy Young Men is Associated with Decreased Leptin Levels, Elevated Ghrelin Levels, and Increased Hunger and Appetite. *Ann Intern Med.* 2004 Dec 7;141(11):846-50.

3. Perlmutter, D. (2013). Grain Brain: The Surprising Truth about Wheat, Carbs, and Sugar--Your Brain's Silent Killers. New York, NY: Little, Brown and Company

4. Lustig, R. H. (2013). Fat Chance: Beating the Odds Against Sugar, Processed Food, Obesity, and Disease. New York, NY: Penguin Group.

5. Ibid.

Chapter 11: Tame the Stress Monster

1. Bjorntorp P, Rosmond R, Obesity and cortisol. *Nutrition*. 2000 Oct;16(10):924-36.

2. Daubenmier J, Kristeller J, Hecht FM, Maninger N, Kuwata M, Jhavier K, Lustig RH, Kemeny M, Karan L, Epel E. Mindfulness Intervention for Stress Eating to Reduce Cortisol and Abdominal Fat among Overweight and Obese Women: An Exploratory Randomized Controlled Study. *Journal of Obesity*. 2011: 651936.

3. Tomiyama AJ, Dallman MF, Epel ES. Comfort Food Is Comforting to Those Most Stressed: Evidence of the Chronic Stress Response Network in High-Stress Women. *Psychoneuroendocrinology* 2011 Nov;36(10):1513-9

4. Ross, J. (2002). The Mood Cure: The 4-Step Program to Take Charge of Your Emotions—Today. New York, NY: Penguin Group

5. Ibid.

Chapter 12: Cook Like Your Great-Grandmother

1. *Fed Up*. Dir. Stephanie Soechtig. Atlas Films. 2014

2. Lustig, R. H. (2013). Fat Chance: Beating the Odds Against Sugar, Processed Food, Obesity, and Disease. New York, NY:

Penguin Group.

3. Ibid.

4. Ibid.

5. Ibid.

6. EWG's Farm Subsidy Database Environmental Working Group (EWG). The United States Farm Subsidy Information http://farm.ewg.org/region.php?fips=00000

7. *Fed Up*. Dir. Stephanie Soechtig. Atlas Films. 2014

8. Egan S. How Well Do You Know Your Food Labels? *New York Times*. May 3, 2016, http://well.blogs.nytimes.com/2016/05/03/how-well-do-you-know-your-food-labels/?_r=0

9. Robinson, J. (2013). Eating on the Wild Side: The Missing Link to Optimum Health. New York, NY: Little, Brown and Company

Chapter 13: Crank Up Your Metabolism

1. Ross, J. (2012). The Diet Cure: The 8-Step Program to Rebalance Your Body Chemistry and End Food Cravings, Weight Gain, and Mood Swings Naturally. New York, NY: Penguin Group.

2. Kolata G. For an Exercise Afterburn, Intensity May be the Key. *The New York Times*. April 18, 2011.

3. *Ibid*.

4. Ross, J. (2012). The Diet Cure: The 8-Step Program to

Rebalance Your Body Chemistry and End Food Cravings, Weight Gain, and Mood Swings Naturally. New York, NY: Penguin Group.

Chapter 14: Keep Moving

1. Lustig, R. H. (2013). Fat Chance: Beating the Odds Against Sugar, Processed Food, Obesity, and Disease. New York, NY: Penguin Group.

2. Ibid.

3. DiSalvo D. How Exercise Makes Your Brain Grow. *Forbes.* Oct. 13, 2013

4. Perlmutter, D. (2013). Grain Brain: The Surprising Truth about Wheat, Carbs, and Sugar--Your Brain's Silent Killers. New York, NY: Little, Brown and Company

5. Ibid.

6. Pedersen BK. The anti-inflammatory effect of exercise: its role in diabetes and cardiovascular disease control. *Essays Biochem* 2006;42:105-17.

7. The University of Aberdeen News, "Want a new body? Get a new 'buddy'" October 4, 2016

Part 5: Where to Begin

Chapter 15: Tips for Transitioning

1. Faunalytics, "How Many Former Vegetarians and Vegans are there?" https://faunalytics.org/how-many-former-vegetarians-and-vegans-are-there/

Index

About the Author

Susan is a Board Certified, Holistic Health Coach and received her training from the Institute for Integrative Nutrition. She began her career in marketing and later became a health coach and writer to fulfill her passion for helping people improve their health and well-being. This is her first book.